A Radiologist's Path

Jason Shames • Lisa Zorn
Kahyun Yoon-Flannery
Editors

A Radiologist's Path

What to Expect after a Radiology Residency

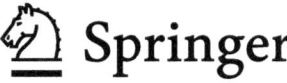
Springer

Editors
Jason Shames
Department of Radiology
Jefferson Health & Thomas Jefferson
University
Philadelphia, PA, USA

Lisa Zorn
Department of Radiology
Jefferson Health & Thomas Jefferson
University
Philadelphia, PA, USA

Kahyun Yoon-Flannery
MD Anderson Cancer Center at Cooper
Cooper Medical School of Rowan
University
Camden, NJ, USA

ISBN 978-3-031-86881-8   ISBN 978-3-031-86882-5   (eBook)
https://doi.org/10.1007/978-3-031-86882-5

Introduction

Finding Your Specialty: Why Radiology Might Be the Perfect Fit

Finding the right specialty can be a daunting task. Even though the road to matriculating as a provider is long, we frequently aren't able to fully experience the various career paths one could venture down during training. Radiology tends to be one of those pathways students get limited exposure to despite its vast interconnectivity and importance to most disciplines. It is the one field an incredibly small number of people leave and a large number cross-train into, and for good reason. It offers some of the most variety in working environments, provides rewarding interactions with both patients and providers, gives access to innovation and research, and has great work-life balance. For those who know they are meant for radiology, we hope this book will help set yourself up for a long and successful career. For those still undecided, we hope this book's glimpse into the field will turn the once-daunting task into one of the easiest decisions you've ever made.

Philadelphia, PA, USA   Jason Shames

Contents

Contributors

Dana Amiraian Department of Radiology, Mayo Clinic, Jacksonville, FL, USA

Rashmi Balasubramanya Department of Radiology, Thomas Jefferson University Hospital, Philadelphia, PA, USA

Jeffrey A. Belair Thomas Jefferson University, Philadelphia, PA, USA

Gilda Boroumand Department of Radiology, Norwalk Hospital, Norwalk, CT, USA

Wilbur Chang Department of Diagnostic and Interventional Radiology, Mid-Atlantic Permanente Medical Group (MAPMG), Rockville, MD, USA

Fatima Iftikhar Chouhdry Department of Breast Imaging, Mount Sinai Health System, Icahn School of Medicine at Mount Sinai, New York, NY, USA

Andrew T. Colucci Department of Radiology, Norwalk Hospital, Norwalk, CT, USA

Tessa S. Cook Department of Radiology, Perelman School of Medicine at the University of Pennsylvania, Philadelphia, PA, USA

Sharon L. D'Souza Tulsa Radiology Associates, Tulsa, OK, USA

Jake A. Gibbons Department of Radiology, Baylor University Medical Center, Dallas, TX, USA

Ekta Gupta Department of Radiology, Zucker School of Medicine at Hofstra Northwell Health, Lake Success, NY, USA

Amy Haberman Department of Radiology, NYU Grossman School of Medicine, New Hyde Park, NY, USA

Theresa Kaufman Department of Radiology, Thomas Jefferson University Hospitals, Philadelphia, PA, USA

Chhavi Kaushik Department of Radiology, Thomas Jefferson University Hospital, Philadelphia, PA, USA

Hamid R. Latifi Department of Radiology, Baylor University Medical Center, Dallas, TX, USA

Ainsley MacLean Department of Diagnostic and Interventional Radiology, Mid-Atlantic Permanente Medical Group (MAPMG), Rockville, MD, USA

Suzanne McElligott Department of Radiology, Zucker School of Medicine at Hofstra Northwell Health, Lake Success, NY, USA

Anne Kathryn Misiura Department of Radiology, Thomas Jefferson University Hospital, Philadelphia, PA, USA

Priya Mody Department of Radiology, University of North Carolina at Chapel Hill, Chapel Hill, NC, USA

Thea Moran MyriadMD Radiology Consulting, LLC, New Orleans, LA, USA

Kristina Nowitzki Department of Radiology, Norwalk Hospital, Norwalk, CT, USA
Specialty Imaging, Danbury, CT, USA

Sophia R. O'Brien Division of Nuclear Medicine Imaging and Therapy, Department of Radiology, University of Pennsylvania, Philadelphia, PA, USA

Austin R. Pantel Division of Nuclear Medicine Imaging and Therapy, Department of Radiology, University of Pennsylvania, Philadelphia, PA, USA

Amit Patel Spouse of a Radiologist, Moorestown, NJ, USA

Ripple S. Patel Department of Radiology, Thomas Jefferson University Hospital, Philadelphia, PA, USA

Lauren C. Pringle Department of Radiology, University of Missouri – Columbia, Columbia, MO, USA

Shashi Ranganath Department of Diagnostic and Interventional Radiology, Mid-Atlantic Permanente Medical Group (MAPMG), Rockville, MD, USA

Evan Rochlis Thomas Jefferson University, Philadelphia, PA, USA

Christopher Roth Jefferson Health & Thomas Jefferson University, Philadelphia, PA, USA

Robyn G. Roth Department of Radiology, Cooper University Hospital, Camden, NJ, USA

Baskaran Sundaram Thomas Jefferson University Hospital, Philadelphia, PA, USA

Pranav Suri University of Missouri – Columbia School of Medicine, Columbia, MO, USA

Jason Shames Department of Radiology, Jefferson Health & Thomas Jefferson University, Philadelphia, PA, USA

Kiran Talekar Thomas Jefferson University, Philadelphia, PA, USA

Satvik Tripathi Department of Radiology, Perelman School of Medicine at the University of Pennsylvania, Philadelphia, PA, USA

Kahyun Yoon-Flannery MD Anderson Cancer Center at Cooper, Cooper Medical School of Rowan University, Camden, NJ, USA

Adam C. Zoga Thomas Jefferson University, Philadelphia, PA, USA

Lisa Zorn Department of Radiology, Jefferson Health & Thomas Jefferson University, Philadelphia, PA, USA

Part I
Training

Chapter 1
Diagnostic Radiology Residency

Thea Moran

Introduction

What is a diagnostic radiologist?

A diagnostic radiologist (DR) is a medical doctor who uses electromagnetic radiation (EMR) to diagnose, and sometimes treat, disease in any organ system. The modalities that use electromagnetic radiation are plain film, ultrasound, CT scan, MRI, and nuclear medicine. Electromagnetic radiation is not harmless to patients, the public, or radiology staff and therefore must be kept at safe levels. Radiologists, as a part of their training, study how each modality creates their respective EMRs to limit radiation exposure while maintaining enough exposure to provide images of sufficient diagnostic quality (I hope you like physics!!!!).

A DR is a "doctor's doctor." Hands-on patient contact is very little compared to, say, internists or surgeons. Instead, the internist or general surgeon has already seen the patient and has formed a differential diagnosis. The DR sometimes helps the referring doctor select the diagnostic test that will give the most necessary diagnostic information while maintaining EMR ALARA (as low as reasonably achievable) levels. Every DR creates a radiology report after evaluating ("reading") the ordered imaging study. The report gives a differential diagnosis that considers both the current and past imaging findings, as well as the history provided by the referrers (histories can be very puny—the bane of every radiologist's existence!)

DRs go through 4 years of residency and require testing to be board certified. This will be discussed later in this chapter. After residency, postgrads can either go into practice or enter a fellowship. Fellowships get into the nitty-gritty of some of

T. Moran (✉)
MyriadMD Radiology Consulting, LLC, New Orleans, LA, USA
e-mail: tmoran@myriadmd.com

© The Author(s), under exclusive license to Springer Nature   3
Switzerland AG 2025
J. Shames et al. (eds.), *A Radiologist's Path*,
https://doi.org/10.1007/978-3-031-86882-5_1

the DR subspecialties, for example, pediatrics or neuroradiology. These will be discussed in later chapters.

I talked about how DRs can sometimes treat disease, but how? Certain subspecialties, such as abdominal, musculoskeletal, and breast imaging, routinely perform procedures to diagnose and treat diseases within their subspecialty's organ system. Interventional radiology (IR), now its own specialty requiring multiple years of both DR and IR training, focuses mainly on procedures to diagnose and treat the patient. The pathways to DR/IR board certification are also discussed in later chapters. Another way DRs can treat patients is via I131 for thyroid cancer. But I'll leave further discussion of that to the nuclear medicine docs.

Pathway to Diagnostic Radiology Training

There is only one pathway to becoming a board-certified DR. All ACGME- and RSPSC-accredited DR residencies require graduation from a medical school that is LCME (if MD) or AOACOCA (if DO) accredited if the school is in the USA. A valid ECFMG certification, and when eligible, a full and unrestricted license to practice medicine in the same US jurisdiction as your ACGME-accredited program is needed if your medical school was from outside of North America.

Internships need to be in direct patient care for a minimum of 36 weeks; a maximum of 2 months of nondirect patient care rotations can occur in DR, IR, or nuclear medicine but must occur in radiology departments with a DR, IR, or nuclear medicine residency program satisfying ACGME requirements. US-based internships need to be completed in an ACGME-accredited, AOA-approved, RCPSC-accredited, or CFPC-accredited program; other programs must have ACGME International Advanced Specialty Accreditation [1]. Your medical school can direct you to their institutional office, which will have further information.

Applying to Programs

Finding a diagnostic radiology program that will be a fit is key; bonus points if you find an internship that is a fit, but that is only a year and the residency is four. I'd start with browsing the ERAS website which will give you the basic info about all participating programs [2]. As of July 2024, there are 185 participating diagnostic radiology programs listed with the Electronic Residency Application Service (ERAS). ERAS streamlines the process, so if I were you, I'd stick with their participating programs. Once you develop a "long list" from the ERAS site, form your "short list" by digging deeper into each of these programs via website searches (ACGME and NRMP websites may be helpful) and word of mouth (mentors come in handy here) because not all pertinent information (i.e., importance of standardized scores/grades/letters/interviews, ACGME accreditation, number of applications received vs available positions, number of applicants interviewed, did they fill their positions in the last few matches, etc.) will be on the ERAS website. It will also be important to dig deeper into whether your programs have more sensitive, off-the-record stuff going on. Examples include anticipated changes in the program's healthcare organization/department/section leadership, mergers/acquisitions of their hospitals, large numbers of staff radiologists coming into or leaving the department, etc. This eliminates any programs that could have a large culture/program shift between interviewing and starting the program, which eliminates any situation creating a very awkward 4 years of training (it's hard enough learning how to be a competent radiologist). You could browse social media groups, Aunt Minnie, blogs, and chatrooms, but I would approach these with caution. I would put the most trust in your mentor, maybe even the dean's office (they are incentivized to ensure you do well because they look good if you look good). And if you see anything on the internet discussing any of your potential programs, run it past one of the above to get their reaction.

Register with ERAS after you have made your final selections. Choose your programs wisely because applying and interviewing gets expensive. ERAS implemented program signaling in 2023 to allow applicants to indicate their interest and intent to match with a particular DR or IR program. During the 2024–2025 match year, applicants were given a total of 12 signals (six gold (most preferred) and six silver (preferred)). Given the many highly qualified candidates applying for a limited number of positions, signaling can give your application an extra boost to secure an interview.

Medical students begin applying early in the fourth year, but don't be shy about getting started early on the application process. The 2024 ERAS Residency Timeline is on the website [3]; this only gives a rough idea of when the ERAS deadlines occur and exact dates change yearly. ERAS participating programs receive applications directly. Most medical schools are ERAS participants; therefore, they will directly submit letters and transcripts to your programs. I personally would confirm with the dean's office that they correctly understand your selected programs and do not rely on technology to do it for you. Choose your DR references early. Choosing references that you have a strong relationship with and preferably know people in your selected programs is most advantageous. It is ok to check with your programs to ensure they received your application and other necessary information. If components of your application are absent, diplomatically proceed to remedy the issue(s). A table/spreadsheet can help organize when things are due and when/if they get submitted.

Interviewing

Programs vary widely in how they perform their interviews; the "basic 411" is provided online, or you can directly reach out to the programs. Being on time, attentive, and looking professional all go without saying. Fair game questions include the following: what are the rotation and call schedules, when will residents be expected to give preliminary reads independently, hospital safety/security, what do DR residents do for their internship year, where do the residents live, what do residents do postgraduation, and what procedures can be expected and to what extent do residents participate in them, opportunities for research/publication. Looking at the interview as a "networking opportunity" is a more positive approach than "I hope I get in." Loyalty reward programs, whether for flights, cars, or hotels, can help cut costs. If you are not part of a loyalty program, sign up for one now and pick one where points don't expire. It's also good to pick one that partners with other loyalty programs, such as Starbucks.

The Match

So…what is "The Match"? The following is a quote from the National Resident Matching Program (NRMP) website [4]:

> The NRMP provides the mechanism through the Registration, Ranking, and Results® (R3®) system for applicants and programs to enter rank order lists of their true preferences. NRMP uses a mathematical algorithm to match applicants and programs to their most preferred ranked choices to make the best possible match for all participants

NRMP is separate from ERAS; therefore, it requires another registration and has another set of deadlines. I provided the 2025 Main Residency Match Applicants Calendar [5] to give an idea of when the deadlines would fall, but I would start checking the relevant calendar by the middle of your third year for the deadlines. As of January 2024, the initial $70 registration fee allows you to list up to 20 programs; after that, there will be supplemental fees [6].

Match lists are submitted after all interviews have been completed. A well-thought-out match list is worth the hard effort that goes into it. Successfully matching is a whole lot easier than going through the supplemental offer and acceptance program (SOAP) (AKA "scrambling"). It is possible to not match in either internship or residency or both residency and internship. Your medical school should be able to help you through this process; however, an ounce of prevention is worth a pound of cure. It is wise to balance the likelihood of matching into a program vs the kind of education you *need* (not *want*) to limit the chances of having to scramble.

Rotation Specifications of DR Residencies

The ACGME educational requirements for diagnostic radiology residencies are extensive and are set forth on their website [7]. The six competencies (patient care, medical knowledge, practice-based learning and improvement, interpersonal and communication skills, professionalism, and systems-based practice) are the cornerstones of any contemporary residency. Residents are required to report their procedural cases to the ACGME Case Log System [8]. There are minimum numbers required for specific procedures [9].

Pathway to Initial Board Certification

A DR resident can take the qualifying core exam after the first 36 months (Fig. 1.1). The qualifying core exam is image rich, computer based, and given twice a year; the 2024 and 2025 timelines show approximate times for important dates [11], but, again, I would check the website during the PGY-4 year for the current dates. The qualifying core exam tests the competency of key concepts in multiple practice domains (including noninterpretive skills, physics, and radioisotope safety). Each domain is listed on the ABR website to show the potential breadth and depth possible for the exam [12]. There are study guides for noninterpretive skills and physics. However, the best exam preparation is consistent, daily image interpretation with subject matter reading.

A DR resident becomes a candidate for the certifying examination about 15 months after residency completion and after passing the qualifying core exam. This examination is also computer based and image dense. Information synthesis, forming a differential diagnosis, and patient management are emphasized in this day-long test. The candidate can pick three modules from different practice areas for their test. Each module will have two levels of difficulty: fundamental and advanced. Pediatric, physics, and radioisotope safety questions will be included in the questions. The fourth module is in Essentials of Diagnostic Radiology and is mandatory. This module includes knowledge that every radiologist should know and will have noninterpretive skills content [13].

For DR residents starting in July 2023 and beyond, the DR certifying exam will be replaced by the new DR oral exam. DR postgraduates will take the oral exam the calendar year after completion of their DR residency. More information as it is updated will be available at the New Diagnostic Radiology Oral Exam site [14].

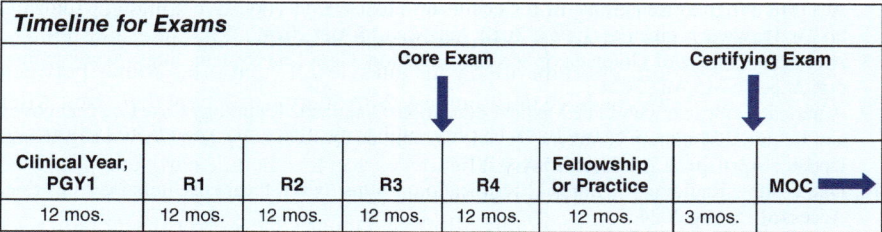

Fig. 1.1 Diagnostic Radiology timeline for exams [10]. (Used with permission of the American Board of Radiology, current as of August 15, 2024)

There are two alternative pathways to board certification: international medical graduate and Holman research alternative pathways. Details can be found on the ABR website [15].

Maintaining Active Board Certification AKA Maintenance of Certification (MOC)

Board eligibility begins immediately after completion of the DR residency and ends 6 years later or at board certification, whichever comes first. DR residents who successful pass all rotations and both the qualifying and certifying exams are granted initial DR board certification. Board certification is a filter universally used by employers during the hiring process, so it is very much to your advantage to have it.

Physicians are required to engage in Maintenance of Certification (MOC) to keep active board certification and your market viability. The MOC process begins immediately after initial board certification. MOC requirements/participation guidelines are on the ABR website [16].

References

1. ACGME Program Requirements for Graduate Medical Education in Diagnostic Radiology, pp 20–22. www.acgme.org. July 1, 2022. Accessed 13 Aug 2024.
2. ERAS® 2024 Participating specialties and programs. ACGME Residency—September Cycle Diagnostic Radiology wwwaamcorg/eras/eras/ Updated July 22, 2024. Accessed 13 Aug 2024.
3. ERAS®. Residency Timeline | Students & Residents. 2024. https://students-residents.aamc.org/eras-tools-and-worksheets-residency-applicants/2024-eras-residency-timeline. Accessed 15 Aug 2024.
4. The Match National Residency Matching Program. Intro to the Match. https://www.nrmp.org/intro-to-the-match/. Accessed 15 Aug 2024.
5. The Match. National Residency Matching Program. Main Residency Match Applicants Calendar. 2024. https://www.nrmp.org/match-calendars/main-residency-applicants/. Accessed 15 Aug 2024.
6. The Match. Intro to the Match. Match Fees https://www.nrmp.org/intro-to-the-match/match-fees/. Accessed 15 Aug 2024.
7. ACGME Program Requirements for Graduate Medical Education in Diagnostic Radiology, pp 23–41. www.acgme.org. July 1, 2022. Accessed 15 Aug 2024.
8. American College of Graduate of Medical Eduction. Case Log System. https://www.acgme.org. Accessed 15 Aug 2024.
9. American College of Graduate Medical Education. Diagnostic Radiology Case Log Categories and Required Minimum Numbers. Review Committee for Radiology. https://www.acgme.org. Updated April 2024. Accessed 15 Aug 2024.
10. Diagnostic Radiology: Initial Certification. https://www.theabr.org/initial-certification. Accessed 15 Aug 2024.
11. American Board of Radiology Exam Dates and Locations. https://www.theabr.org/diagnostic-radiology/calendar. Accessed 15 Aug 2024.

12. American Board of Radiology. Initial Certification for Diagnostic Radiology. Qualifying (Core) Exam. Preparing for the Qualifying (Core) Exam. https://www.theabr.org/diagnostic-radiology/initial-certification/core-exam/studying-core-exam. Accessed 15 Aug 2024.
13. American Board of Radiology. Initial Certification in Diagnostic Radiology. Certifying Exam. https://www.theabr.org/diagnostic-radiology/initial-certification/core-exam/certifying-exam.
14. American Board of Radiology. Initial Certification for Diagnostic Radiology. News from the ABR. New Diagnostic Radiology Oral Exam. https://www.theabr.org/news/new-diagnostic-radiology-oral-exam. Accessed 15 Aug 2024.
15. American Board of Radiology. Initial Certification for Diagnostic Radiology. Alternative Pathways. https://www.theabr.org/diagnostic-radiology/initial-certification.alternate-pathways. Accessed 15 Aug 2024.
16. American Board of Radiology. Continuing Certification (MOC) Participation Guidelines. https://www.theabr.org/diagnostic-radiology/maientenance-or-certification. Accessed 15 Aug 2024.

Chapter 2
Integrated Interventional Radiology Residency

Thea Moran

Is IR for me?

So…you want to become an interventional radiologist? Perhaps, you thought IR was cool after reading about a celebrity who benefited from an IR procedure. [1] Or maybe one of your colleagues saw an IR procedure done and it lit a fire under them? Maybe one of your attendings who knows you thought you might be a good fit? All of these scenarios are great ways to become interested in IR, but how do you figure out if it really is for you? Probably, the best way to see if IR is a good fit is to spend time in the IR suite, watch procedures, participate as appropriate, talk to and observe the attendings/residents, and don't be shy about asking questions. Great questions to ask would be "what do you like/not like about IR," "what got you interested in IR," "what are the job possibilities after IR training (including practice types (general vs specialized jobs)), and how easy is the job search, lifestyle, etc.). Attendings will be able to the give a "big picture" perspective, while residents will have more bandwidth; residents will be better able to give a perspective on training, applying, and interviewing, so get both perspectives if you can. As a medical student, performing either a dedicated IR elective or a radiology elective with special focus on IR is even better. Look into externships for IR electives if an elective is not offered at your institution. It would be wise to perform any IR electives through an ACGME-accredited IR program.

T. Moran (✉)
MyriadMD Radiology Consulting, LLC, New Orleans, LA, USA
e-mail: tmoran@myriadmd.com

© The Author(s), under exclusive license to Springer Nature Switzerland AG 2025
J. Shames et al. (eds.), *A Radiologist's Path*,
https://doi.org/10.1007/978-3-031-86882-5_2

Pathways to Getting IR Training

In 1953, Ivar Seldinger developed a percutaneous technique which resulted in the ability to perform vascular, and other, diagnostic, or therapeutic interventions without the need for surgical cut down [2]. In 1964, Charles Dotter published a case series describing significant clinical and radiologic improvement in vascular patients post-transluminal catheter dilation [3], something now known as angioplasty. The diagnostic and therapeutic possibilities, vascular and otherwise, which evolved from these two techniques are phenomenal. They are so phenomenal that the current IR skill set and fund of knowledge that a competent IR is expected to have are well past what a board-certified diagnostic radiologist should be expected to know. In 2012, the American Board of Medical Specialties (ABMS) formally recognized IR as a distinct specialty. One IR training pathway is through an independent IR residency which first requires completion of a diagnostic radiology residency; Chap. 20 discusses this program type in detail. The second pathway is the integrated IR residency which is where both diagnostic and interventional radiology training are provided within one program. Medical students deciding early that they want an IR career most commonly select this pathway. *This chapter will focus on the second IR training pathway, but you are encouraged to also read Chap. 19 because there is information overlap between the chapters.* International medicine graduates or transfers from other programs are not discussed in this chapter; I encourage these candidates to contact Postgraduate Medical Education affairs at the Society of Interventional Radiology (SIR) (gme@sirweb.org) for more information. Figure 2.1 lays out the differences between the IR pathways.

All ACGME- or RCPSC-accredited IR residencies will require an internship before starting IR training. There are requirements for your ACGME-accredited internship year [4]. Your medical school can direct you to the office that has that information.

Year	Traditional Pathway Offered thru 6/30/202	Integrated IR Residency	Independent IR Residency Offered starting 7/1/2020	Independent IR Residency with ESIR Offered starting 7/1/2020
PGY-1	1 year of ACGME-accredited non-radiology clinical training (internship year)			
PGY-2	Diagnostic Radiology Residency	3 years of diagnostic radiology training	Diagnostic Radiology Residency	Diagnostic Radiology Residency with Early Specialization in Interventional Radiology (ESIR) included
PGY-3				
PGY-4				
PGY-5		2 years of IR training		
PGY-6	1 year of IR Fellowship		2 years of Independent IR Residency	1 year of Independent IR Residency
PGY-7	N/A	N/A		N/A
Total Years of Training	6	6	7	6

Fig. 2.1 Interventional radiology training pathways [5]. Used with permission of the American Board of Radiology, current as of January 2024

Applying to Programs

First, you need to find an integrated IR residency that you think will be a fit. Most integrated IR residency programs participate in the Electronic Residency Application Service (ERAS), so perusing the ERAS website will get you the basic 411 on the currently listed 97 integrated IR residencies who use ERAS [6]; not all programs use ERAS, but it's probably easier to stick with the ones that do. I suggest that you do your own research on the programs that interest you because not all relevant information will be on the ERAS website, i.e., importance a program gives to standardized scores/grades/letters/interviews, ACGME-accreditation, how many applications received/available positions, how many applicants are interviewed, did they fill their positions in the match, etc. After you've done that, ask around to see if there is any off-the-record information about your programs of interest that may influence your decision, i.e., are there any anticipated upcoming changes in your program's healthcare organization/department/section leadership, mergers/acquisitions of hospitals, anticipated large numbers of staff radiologists coming or leaving the department, etc. This eliminates any programs that could have a large culture/program shift between when you interviewed and when you start the program because otherwise, it could be a very, very long 5 yrs. Hopefully, you have selected a mentor who can help ferret out some information.

After you pick your program "short list", register with ERAS. Choose your programs wisely because applying and interviewing gets expensive. Medical students begin applying early in the fourth year; the earlier you get started on the application process, the better. The 2024 ERAS Residency Timeline is on the website [7]; this only gives a rough idea of when the ERAS deadlines occur but exact dates change yearly. ERAS-participating programs receive applications directly. Most medical schools are ERAS participants; therefore, they will directly submit letters and transcripts to your programs; I, personally, would confirm with the dean's office that they correctly understand your selected programs and not rely on technology to do it for you. Choose your IR references early. It is most advantageous to choose references that you have a strong relationship with and who know people in your selected programs, but, if they don't know people in the programs, it's not a deal breaker. It is ok to check with your programs to make sure they received your application and other necessary information. If components of your application are absent, diplomatically proceed to remedy the issue(s). I would use the table/spreadsheet suggestion I put in Chap. 19 under the same section.

Interviewing

Programs will vary widely in how they perform their interviews; details are provided as per "the basic 411" described above and/or calling the programs. Being on time and attentive, as well as looking professional, goes without saying. Questions asking about rotation and call schedules, whether call is in-house or from home, hospital safety/security, what have prior integrated IR residents done for their internship year, where do the residents live, what do residents do after graduation, procedure mix, opportunities for research/publication, are all fair game. Looking at the interview as a "networking opportunity" is a more positive approach than "I hope I get in.". If you really want to do IR, sooner or later, you will, so relax. IRs tend to know and engage with each other a lot, so do what you can to exude warmth and a love for collaboration (especially with fellow interviewees). Loyalty reward programs, whether they are for flights, cars, or hotels, can help cut costs. If you are not part of a loyalty program, sign up for one now and pick one where points don't expire. It's also good to pick one that partners with other loyalty programs. For example, I belong to both Delta and Starbucks loyalty programs, neither of which have points that expire and when I get a latte, not only do I get points to use toward a free latte later, but I also get Delta SkyMiles points (not many, but some). Do it enough times and you can eventually treat yourself, at least in part, to a nice, well-earned trip.

The Match

So…what is this "rank" business and what is the best way to do it? The following is a quote from the National Resident Matching Program (NRMP) website [8]:

> The NRMP provides the mechanism through the Registration, Ranking, and Results® (R3®) system for applicants and programs to enter rank order lists of their true preferences. NRMP uses a mathematical algorithm to match applicants and programs to their most preferred ranked choices to make the best possible match for all participants

NRMP is separate from ERAS; therefore, it requires another registration and has another set of deadlines. I provided the 2024 Main Residency Match Applicants Calendar [9] to give an idea when the deadlines would fall but I would start checking the relevant calendar by the middle of your third year for the deadlines. As of January 2024, the initial $70 registration fee allows you to list up to 20 programs; after that, there will be supplemental fees [10].

Match lists are submitted after all interviews have been completed. A well-thought-out match list is worth its weight in gold. Successfully matching is a whole lot easier than going through the supplemental offer and acceptance program (SOAP) (AKA "scrambling"). It is possible to not match in either internship or residency or in both residency and internship. Your medical school should be able to help you through this process; however, an ounce of prevention is worth a pound of cure. It is wise to balance the likelihood of matching into a program vs the kind of education you *need* (not *want*) to limit the chances of having to scramble.

Rotation Specifications of Integrated IR Residencies

The first 36 months of an integrated IR residency is in diagnostic radiology and the subsequent 24 months are in IR. The program requirements for the first 36 months are the same as for the diagnostic radiology residency (see Chap. 1). Because most starting integrated IR residents have no practical IR experience where competencies are recorded, there are many program requirements for the 24 months of IR [11]. Residents are required to report the cases they participate in through the ACGME case log mechanism [12].

Pathway to Initial Board Certification

An integrated IR resident can take the qualifying core exam after the first 36 months. It is the same exam that is taken by the diagnostic radiology residents. The qualifying core exam is image rich, computer based, and given twice a year; the 2024 and 2025 timelines show approximate times for important dates [13], but, again, I would check the website during the PGY-4 year for the current dates. The qualifying core exam tests competency of key concepts in multiple practice domains (including noninterpretive skills, physics, and radioisotope safety). Each domain, including noninterpretive skills and physics, has a study guide on the ABR website [14]. The overviews only give guidance, with the best preparation being consistent, daily image interpretation and subject matter reading.

An integrated IR resident becomes a candidate for the certifying examination after residency completion and after passing the qualifying core exam. The certifying examination tests medical judgment. There are two components to the certifying examination: computer based and oral. The computer-based exam is 4 hours long and the oral exam is 3 hours long; the exams are given on separate dates. The computer-based exam has two modules: essentials of diagnostic radiology and interventional radiology. The oral exam has four 30-minute sessions where the candidate discusses IR cases with a specific examiner dedicated to each 30-min session. Study guides for all portions of the certifying exam are available on the ABR website [15].

Maintaining Active Board Certification AKA Maintenance of Certification (MOC)

Board eligibility begins immediately after completion of the IR residency and ends 6 years later or at board certification, whichever comes first. Integrated IR residents who pass both the qualifying and certifying exams, and successfully complete all rotations, are granted initial DR/IR board certification. Board certification is the holy grail for any physician; it is a filter universally used by employers during the hiring process. Physicians are required to engage in Maintenance of Certification (MOC) to keep the board certification active. MOC has been the subject of much debate but, regardless, it is a hoop that currently needs to be jumped through to stay competitive in the job market. The MOC process begins immediately after initial board certification. MOC requirements/participation guidelines can be found on the ABR website [16].

References

1. CNN.com. Rice 'resting comfortably' after surgery. November 19, 2004. 2004. https://www.cnn.com/2004/. Accessed 17 Feb 2023.
2. Seldinger SI. Catheter replacement of the needle in percutaneous arteriography: a new technique. Acta Radiol. 1953;39(5):368–76. https://doi.org/10.1080/02841850802133386.
3. Dotter CT, Judkins MP. Transluminal treatment of arteriosclerotic obstruction description of a new technic and a preliminary report of its application. Circulation. 1964;30(5):654–70. https://doi.org/10.1161/01.CIR.30.5.654.
4. ACGME Program Requirements for Graduate Medical Education in Interventional Radiology, pp 25–26. www.acgme.org. July 1, 2022. Accessed 18 Jan 2024.
5. Interventional radiology: initial certification. interventional radiology training pathways. https://www.theabr.org/. Updated December 18, 2023. Accessed 13 Jan 2024.
6. ERAS®. Participating specialties and programs. ACGME Residency—September Cycle. Interventional Radiology – Integrated. 2024. www.aamc.org/eras/eras/. Updated September 12, 2023. Accessed 13 Jan 2024.
7. ERAS®. Residency Timeline | Students & Residents. 2024 https://students-residents.aamc.org/eras-tools-and-worksheets-residency-applicants/2024-eras-residency-timeline. Accessed 13 Jan 2024.
8. The Match National Residency Matching Program. Intro to the match. https://www.nrmp.org/intro-to-the-match/. Accessed 13 Jan 2024.
9. The Match. National residency matching program. Main residency match applicants calendar. 2024. https://www.nrmp.org/match-calendars/main-residency-applicants/. Accessed 13 Jan 2024.
10. The Match. Intro to the match. Match Fees https://www.nrmp.org/intro-to-the-match/match-fees/. Accessed 19 Jan 2024.
11. ACGME program requirements for graduate medical education in interventional radiology, pp 30–36. www.acgme.org. July 1, 2022. Accessed 19 Jan 2024.
12. American College of Graduate Medical Education. Guidelines for tracking interventional radiology patient care and procedural experiences. Review committee for radiology. https://www.acgme.org. Updated December 2017. Accessed 13 Jan 2024.
13. American Board of Radiology Exam Dates and Locations. https://www.theabr.org/interventional-radiology/calendar. Accessed 13 Jan 2024.
14. American Board of Radiology. Initial certification in interventional radiology. Qualifying (Core) Exam. Preparing for the Qualifying (Core) Exam. https://www.theabr.org/interventional-radiology/initial-certification/core-exam/studying-core-exam. Accessed 14 Jan 2024.
15. American Board of Radiology. Initial certification in interventional radiology. IR/DR certifying exam. Studying for the Exam. https://www.theabr.org/interventional-radiology/initial-certification/irdr-certifying-exam. Accessed 14 Jan 2024.
16. American Board of Radiology. Continuing certification (moc) participation guidelines. https://www.theabr.org/interventional-radiology/maintenance-of-certification/moc-participation-guidelines. Accessed 14 Jan 2024.

Chapter 3
Combined Diagnostic Radiology and Nuclear Medicine

Sophia R. O'Brien and Austin R. Pantel

Nuclear medicine (NM) is a diverse, exciting, and rapidly evolving patient-facing field.

Nuclear medicine physicians read diagnostic studies for medical and surgical patients of all ages, collaborate with many different medical specialties, and even treat patients with radiopharmaceutical therapy.

In the United States, there are five American Council for Graduate Medical Education (ACGME) approved pathways for nuclear medicine (NM) training [1, 2]:

Type of NM training	Years to complete (after intern year)	Eligible for diagnostic radiology ABR[a] certification?	Eligible for NM specialty[b] certification?
Diagnostic radiology (DR) residency: all DR trainees participate in at least 4 months of NM training during their general DR training	4 years	Yes	No
Combined nuclear medicine-diagnostic radiology residency	5 years	Yes	Yes
16-month pathway: nuclear medicine fellowship integrated into diagnostic radiology residency	4 years	Yes	Yes
Nuclear medicine/radiology fellowship: a one-year fellowship following DR residency	5 years	Yes	Yes

(continued)

S. R. O'Brien (✉) · A. R. Pantel
Division of Nuclear Medicine Imaging and Therapy, Department of Radiology,
University of Pennsylvania, Philadelphia, PA, USA
e-mail: Sophia.Obrien@pennmedicine.upenn.edu

© The Author(s), under exclusive license to Springer Nature Switzerland AG 2025
J. Shames et al. (eds.), *A Radiologist's Path*,
https://doi.org/10.1007/978-3-031-86882-5_3

Type of NM training	Years to complete (after intern year)	Eligible for diagnostic radiology ABR[a] certification?	Eligible for NM specialty[b] certification?
Nuclear medicine residency: a completely separate residency from DR	3 years	No	Yes

[a]ABR = American Board of Radiology
[b]NM Specialty Certification can be obtained from the ABR or from the American Board of Nuclear medicine (ABNM). These different certification pathways have different requirements, which may not be fulfilled by each training pathway

This chapter describes NM training obtained in combination with DR residency, briefly discussing exposure to NM obtained in all DR residencies but focusing on the combined nuclear medicine-diagnostic radiology residencies (5-year programs) and the 16-month nuclear medicine fellowships integrated into diagnostic residency (4-year programs).

For discussion of nuclear medicine fellowship (an additional year of training after completion of intern year and a 4-year diagnostic radiology residency), please see Chap. 17 of this book. Nuclear medicine residency is a separate residency from diagnostic radiology and will not be discussed in this book.

NM Training During Typical DR Residency

Nuclear medicine training is a required component of diagnostic radiology residency in the United States, with a minimum of 4 months of NM experience obtained during a resident's four-year DR residency. Completion of NM training during DR residency allows graduates to practice nuclear medicine (read single-photon emission computed tomography [SPECT], positron emission tomography [PET], planar studies, and cardiac nuclear medicine studies) under their board certification from the American Board of Radiology (ABR) [3]. Diagnostic radiology residents may obtain enough nuclear medicine training during their DR residency to apply to be an authorized user and to be able to prescribe radioactive iodine, but this is residency program specific. If you are interested in becoming an authorized user, you should keep this in mind when looking at diagnostic radiology residencies. Trainees *do not* gain enough training during typical DR residency to sit for nuclear specific board certification offered from the ABR (ABR-CAQ) or American Board of Nuclear Medicine (ABNM) nor can they prescribe parenteral radiopharmaceutical therapy (e.g., Lu-177 PSMA therapy for metastatic castrate-resistant prostate cancer, Lu-177 Dotatate for neuroendocrine tumor, among others).

Combined Nuclear Medicine-Diagnostic Radiology Residency

There are a few combined Nuclear Medicine-Diagnostic Radiology residencies in the United States that take 5 years to complete (after intern year). Applicants apply to these programs during their fourth year of medical school and match into a combined NM-DR spot rather than a typical DR residency. There are three active combined nuclear medicine-diagnostic radiology residency programs at the time of this publication (University of California Davis, Stanford, and Johns Hopkins), each accepting one resident per year. The specifics of these programs differ but either include a full year of dedicated NM training first followed by 4 years of DR residency (which often include additional dedicated NM clinical and/or research time) or 4 years of DR residency followed by 1 year of NM training (similar to typical DR residency followed by a NM fellowship). A certain number of radionuclide therapies are required during training but differ by program and by which NM certification (ABR or ABNM) trainees plan to take.

The AMA FREIDA search engine (freida.ama-assn.org) is a good resource for searching for these residency programs.

16-Month Integrated Pathway: NM Fellowship During DR Residency

There are multiple 16-month integrated nuclear radiology fellowship programs which are embedded within a four-year DR training program (as of 2018, 9 DR programs reported offering the 16-month pathway) [4]. As stated before, all DR residents complete 4 months of nuclear medicine training during residency, so the 16-month pathway represents an additional 12 months of dedicated nuclear medicine training (of which four months may be in a "related field," up to the discretion of the DR program director) [5]. Of note, programs that offer a 16-month integrated pathway do not necessarily have to offer a traditional fellowship program.

Application to these integrated fellowships occurs after a trainee has already matched to that particular institution's DR residency, often within their first or second year of DR training. If you are interested in this pathway, be sure to determine if this is offered at the residency programs you are applying to/interviewing at and ask questions about it on your interview day.

The 16 months of NM training do not need to happen consecutively. Many of these programs are often designed such that trainees complete typical DR training for the first three years of their DR residency, often with some additional NM time, with a focus on NM during the majority of their R4 year.

Additionally, 16-month integrated fellows are required to participate in a minimum number of radionuclide therapies:

- Ten cases of oral I-131 NaI less than or equal to 33 mCi.
- Five cases of oral I-131 NaI greater than 33 mCi.

– Five cases of parenteral radionuclide therapies (i.e., I-131 MIBG, Lu-177 Dotatate, and Lu-177 PSMA).

Graduates of an integrated 16-month training in NM are eligible for diagnostic radiology certification by the ABR as well as NM specific certification, either by the ABR or ABNM pending the specifics of their training program. They may then pursue another radiology fellowship the year after graduation, obtaining two full fellowships in the time a typical DR trainee obtains one.

Finding a Residency That Aligns with Your Values and Goals

Besides the logistics of the application process and timing of training, those interested in nuclear medicine training should identify their educational and professional goals to the best of their abilities and try to determine which programs align with those goals.

Like all medical training, location and proximity to family and friends should be considered. Additionally, your ideal job characteristic will influence the priority you place on certain aspects of training. Do you want to work in private practice, academics, a hybrid practice, or a VA? Do you want your job to include teaching, research, advocacy, and/or leadership roles? Do you want to look for a job in the same institution as your residency training or do you want to take your learning from residency to a different institution? There are no right or wrong answers, and no answer is set in stone, but these questions will help you work backward to determine the type and location desired for residency training.

When looking at the specifics of the nuclear medicine training portion of residency, there are many questions to consider. How many combined or integrated residents are accepted on average per year? Does the program tend to fill its slots or are there recent years without a resident in the NM training program? Does the program have other pathways, such as a dedicated nuclear medicine fellowship, and how do the different pathways align and interact?

NM Diagnostic Training

A strong NM program should provide training and experience in adult general nuclear medicine and positron emission tomography (PET), pediatric general nuclear medicine and PET (at the same institution or via a collaborative agreement with a nearby children's hospital), nuclear cardiology, and radiopharmaceutical therapy. As new PET radiotracers receive FDA approval, strong programs will include these tracers in their everyday workflow. Current common adult PET radiotracers used clinically include 18F-FDG (still the workhorse of PET imaging), Cu-54- and Ga-68-DOTATATE imaging for neuroendocrine tumors, F-18- and

Ga-68-PSMA imaging for prostate cancer, and 18F-FES for metastatic/recurrent estrogen receptor positive breast cancer. Pediatric imaging studies include both PET/CT and PET/MRI with 18F-FDG as well as many other radiotracers depending on an institution's historical experience, research interests, and patient population.

Radiopharmaceutical Therapy

Radiopharmaceutical therapy training is not required for DR residents' required NM training during residency. However, NM-DR combined residencies and NM integrated fellowships require classroom training and experience in administering radiopharmaceutical therapy, including low and high doses of oral I-131 and a variety of parenteral radiopharmaceuticals (2). Current common IV radiopharmaceuticals include Lutetium-177 DOTATATE ("Lutathera") for metastatic neuroendocrine tumor, Lu-177 PSMA ("Pluvicto") for metastatic prostate cancer, Radium-223 ("Xofigo") for painful bone-dominant metastatic prostate cancer, and I-131 MIBG for advanced pheochromocytoma/paraganglioma in adults and neuroblastoma in children (note is made that in January 2023 the clinical formulation of I-131 MIBG "Azedra" no is longer be available, affecting patient care and NM training). Not all NM divisions will offer all therapies, and some may offer additional research therapies. Identifying the types of therapies offered and the volume of therapy patients seen by the division will give you insight into the patient populations you will be working with and your expected comfort with radiopharmaceutical therapy by the time of graduation.

Didactics

Well-established NM fellowship programs will have dedicated didactics for nuclear medicine residents/integrated fellows and often case conferences and journal clubs as well. Didactics are required to become authorized users, with the length of didactics explicitly specified to each classification. An integrated training program may also have teaching opportunities for fellows such as resident lecture, resident board review, NM fellow lecture/case conference, or even medical student teaching.

Specific NM Responsibilities

This section likely does not apply to DR residents not pursuing additional dedicated training.

NM-DR combined residents and integrated NM fellows may have nuclear medicine-specific call duties on nights or weekends.

Nuclear medicine physicians often lead radiology review of a multitude of tumor boards, but unlike other radiology specialties, NM/NR physicians can contribute to tumor boards as treating physicians for diseases treated with radiopharmaceutical therapy in NM therapy clinic. NM-DR residents and integrated nuclear fellows often prepare and present the tumor board imaging cases with mentorship by NM faculty. The specific tumor board trainees will be exposed to and the number of tumor board fellows are expected to lead per week or per month will vary by fellowship.

Fellowships may provide academic time during which fellows can prepare for tumor boards and/or nuclear medicine clinic and work on scholarly projects. The amount of academic time, if any, will vary by program and sometimes by year pending the number of fellows in that year's cohort.

Other Considerations

Depending on your career interests, other considerations may include research opportunities (bench, translational, and clinical), leadership opportunities, and amount of mentorship/sponsorship provided by NM faculty.

Conclusion

Nuclear medicine is a dynamic and patient-facing field currently evolving at a rapid pace. The amount of patient contact can vary and may be tailored on an individual basis. New imaging radiotracers and therapy radiopharmaceuticals introduced in recent years are truly changing the field, and additional developments are likely right on the horizon. Nuclear medicine physicians provide diagnostic reads for a variety of nuclear imaging studies, serve as important consultants in multidisciplinary tumor boards, and function as the treating physician for multiple patient populations seeking radiopharmaceutical therapy. Your career goals will determine which of the factors described above are most important in your future NM training and whether you want to pursue additional dedicated NM training beyond that already included in all DR residencies in the United States. Word of mouth is also a very important method of collecting information about a program—your residency institution's NM faculty can often help identify which NM programs would be a good fit for you.

Best of luck, you will be great!

References

1. Arevalo-Perez J, Paris M, Graham MM, Osborne JR. A Perspective of the Future of Nuclear Medicine Training and Certification. Semin Nucl Med. 2016;46(1):88–96.
2. American Board of Nuclear Medicine. Training requirements for the ABNM ceritfying examination. 2023. https://www.abnm.org/exam/training-requirements/. Accessed 1 July 2023.
3. Oates ME. Integrated residency training pathways of the future: diagnostic radiology, nuclear radiology, nuclear medicine, and molecular imaging. J Am Coll Radiol JACR. 2012;9(4):239–44.
4. Harolds JA. Survey of Programs About the ABR 16-Month Nuclear Radiology Pathway for Diagnostic Radiology Residents. J Nucl Med. 2018 Feb;59(2):16N–7N.
5. 16-month Pathway to specialty certification in diagnostic radiology and subspecialty certification in nuclear radiology. The American Board of Radiology. (2023, September 21). https://www.theabr.org/diagnostic-radiology/subspecialties/nuclear-radiology/16-month-pathway.

Chapter 4
Radiology Residency Application

Sharon L. D'Souza and Fatima Iftikhar Chouhdry

Congratulations!! It's the home stretch—you have completed more than half of medical school, you're working through the USMLE steps, and now, you're looking ahead to the next phase of your career. So, you have decided to pursue radiology? WONDERFUL. Excellent choice. Welcome to a challenging, innovative, and always interesting specialty. As "the doctor's doctor," you will have a hand in the care of almost, if not every, person that walks into the hospital. As the imaging expert, you will routinely be consulted by your colleagues in virtually all other specialties. And you will truly be making a difference in the lives of countless patients.

What Makes a Good Candidate?

More often than not, the first exposure a program has to a candidate is their written application. As such, it needs to convey the qualities typically sought after in a residency program. For example, poor grammar or spelling errors in a personal statement seem careless and bring into question your attention to detail and ability to create quality reports for imaging examinations. Usage of correct terminology is also important. Words matter. You are not now, nor have you ever been, in "provider school." The term "provider," besides having unfortunate origins, is deliberately utilized by administration and special interest groups in order to falsely equate individuals with vastly different levels of training and confuse the public. You are a

S. L. D'Souza
Tulsa Radiology Associates, Tulsa, OK, USA

F. I. Chouhdry (✉)
Department of Breast Imaging, Mount Sinai Health System, Icahn School of Medicine at Mount Sinai, New York, NY, USA
e-mail: Fatima.Chouhdry@mountsinai.org

© The Author(s), under exclusive license to Springer Nature Switzerland AG 2025
J. Shames et al. (eds.), *A Radiologist's Path*,
https://doi.org/10.1007/978-3-031-86882-5_4

medical student, you are training to become a physician, and you are applying for a specialized residency; the words you choose in your written and verbal communication need to reflect that.

While your picture doesn't need to be professionally done, it does need to look like you and be fairly recent. I would suggest not using a candid from a party or one of you in a cap and gown from your college graduation (and before you ask—yes, I've seen both).

A Strong Personal Statement Why do you want to be a radiologist? If you can't answer this question effectively, you need to stop and reassess your course of action. Head back to the drawing board and figure out your "why."

Letters of Recommendation Quality is far more important than quantity. Ask people who know you well and can write personalized, positive letters. A lukewarm or even slightly negative letter can quickly call into question an applicant's desirability. Try to have at least one letter from a radiologist.

We've talked about the importance of words, but what about actions? How do we know you truly understand what being a radiologist day in and day out entails that you are not basing your decision on some faulty preconceived notion crafted together from sentiments of physicians in other specialties or perhaps seen on medical tv shows? I've never jumped up and down in my bathrobe yelling "MY machines!!!" like the ever-elusive radiologist on Scrubs. If someone has not made a concerted effort to get involved, to seek out available opportunities, that's a concern and will be asked about. If radiology is an elective at your medical school, make sure you take it. If not, show some initiative and create your own opportunities. For example, talk to a radiologist—we're pretty cool people! Often, if they know you're truly interested, they may allow you to observe during your time off, assist on projects, with research, etc. Attend a radiology specific conference—even better, try to present a poster! Join a radiology group. If you're truly interested in radiology as a lifelong profession, then your CV needs to illustrate that.

Is there is a specific residency program you want to attend? If so, try to arrange a sub-internship, try to do a rotation there before your interview, and use that opportunity to make a good impression; show them what kind of resident you will be. Not only is it a great way to "try before you buy" and get a feel for the culture of the institution, but it shows that you're serious about the specialty and the program.

The Interview

You have made it to the long-awaited interview; now is your time to shine! Half the battle is making it to this point, so be proud of your accomplishments. This means you have already made the cut regarding grades, personal statement, and letters of recommendation. Everything you have worked for thus far has led up to this moment. Be yourself; this is your opportunity to let the program know what draws you to radiology and why you would excel at their institution.

This part of the process is truly about the best "fit" for you and the program to which you are applying. A happy resident makes for a happy program; these people will become like your family. You often spend more time in the hospital than at home, so you want to ensure that your choice is correct, mainly because it can affect your mental and physical health. If you feel good, you will do good. This is one of those long-term relationships that should bring you a sense of fulfillment and contribute to your well-being.

Interviews can be expensive if they involve going on-site to the program and not meeting virtually. You have to factor in the cost of travel, lodging, meals, and numerous other things that may come up for each interview. It doesn't hurt to ask the program coordinator if there are discounted rates for interviewees at the local hotels near the program. Many times, there will be; you just have to ask! Stay organized regarding planning dates for the interview and scheduling all the traveling because interview season can be very hectic. And, also, be nice to the people you meet on the interview trail. They are in this just like you and have worked just as hard. They will become your colleagues in the future, and you might match with them to the same program and have to work with them. If your program offers a preinterview dinner the night before, be conscious of your interactions with your fellow interviewees and current residents. First impressions really can make a difference. For example, becoming inebriated the night before an interview dinner is generally discouraged and in poor form. Save your celebrations for Match Day!

Knowledge truly is power; the more you know about and prepare for the interview, the more comfortable you will feel. Look at each interview day as "Game Day" and have a "Game Plan." Know how you will get to and from the interview site, factoring in transportation and traffic, if any. It is best to be at least 15 minutes early to the interview as it gives you a buffer to freshen up or take a minute to relax before beginning the interview day. Make sure your suit is ironed and laid out the night before. Do not wear distracting clothing/prints/colors because that is not what you have come to be judged on. You want the interviewer to decide if you will be an asset to their program, not why you chose to wear a neon green suit. Wear comfortable shoes because most interviews involve a touring portion, including walking significant distances through the facility. The main point is: look professional and be comfortable.

Look up the program beforehand and know who you are interviewing with, if provided. If they are known in the field because of their research or publications, then it is best to be familiar with them as they come up as a topic of discussion. As a resident, I served on the interview committee and listened to what my attendings were looking for in our applicants. Often, it came down to "Can I make conversation with this person? Will I be able to sit down with them for most of the day?" Be ready for the fundamental questions of "So why radiology, and why this program?" but also be prepared for questions geared to get to know you better as an applicant. Some of these questions may ask about the most recent book you read, the most recent television show you enjoyed, or your hobbies. Other questions may be about your CV, which brings me to my next point: know yourself. Read your CV before-hand and make sure you can support everything you have put on there. All the proj-ects, publications, and activities you have listed on there are fair game for questions. It should go without saying but do not be a liar. No one likes a liar, and it looks ridiculous to defend yourself when caught.

Most importantly, practice. Practice interviewing with a friend or family member or talking to yourself in the mirror. Sometimes, answers sound better in your head and may seem silly when you say them out loud. There is nothing wrong with prac-ticing; by the end of your interview season, you will be a pro!

Game Day: Ok, you made it. You arrived early looking fresh in your suit, other interviewees are filing in, and you are seconds away from a panic attack. Just kid-ding. Breathe. You have made it this far; you got this. Introduce yourself, thank your interviewer for the opportunity, and be the star you already know you are. At the end of the interview day, keep the itinerary sheet you were likely handed at the start of the day. This should have the names of the people you interviewed and their contact information. Make sure you at least have the email addresses of those you encoun-tered on your interview day to send them a follow-up thank you email. Some say a handwritten note is more thoughtful, but an email can do the job just fine. If emails are not provided, then go with the mailing route, but the point is to send a thank you note to show your gratitude for being invited to interview. It may set you apart and secure your position with that program.

Whew, That's Over: What Next?

Keep in mind, many of your interviewers may be from a different generation. Back when I interviewed, I remember being told to send thank you notes; I honestly still routinely do this for every gift, dinner party, etc. While it may not be the current expectation and I don't personally receive many these days, I can't help but remem-ber the interviewees that do make the effort to send a note of thanks. It doesn't take much time, and this small old-fashioned sign of appreciation will be remembered long after you send it and will undoubtedly be seen in a positive light.

After the interview day, list your likes and dislikes regarding the program. Do this immediately after your interview because the day's happenings will be fresh in your mind. Is there something you enjoyed about that day? Anything that you saw as a red flag? Write it all down. This will serve you well when putting together your rank list for Match Day. A helpful next thing to do when you get home is write the program's name on a Post-it note and put that note on your mirror. As your inter-view season progresses, you will end up with more and more Post-its on your mir-ror, which you can arrange based on how you felt about each program; the placement of the Post-its will change after each interview. In doing this, you are making a preliminary rank order list which ultimately helps you make your official list for the Match.

Chapter 5
The Match Process

Fatima Iftikhar Chouhdry

You have finally finished the long season of interviews and are ready to make significant life decisions. At this point, you have hopefully gone through the pros and cons of each program you have interviewed at and come up with a rough list of how you would like to rank them. This is when you need to decide what is most important to you about where you will end up for the next few years. So many factors are going into this decision, like program location, academic vs. community, program size, and probably most important, where you felt most at home. You have a lot of riding on this decision, but trust the process; this is the homestretch!

You will need to register with NRMP, the National Resident Matching Program. The standard registration deadline is January 31; to keep up with the Match calendar, it is best to become familiar with the NRMP website, as many updates, checklists, and frequently asked questions about the process are available there.

Radiology residency is four years, but with the addition of your intern year, it lasts a total of five years (your first year of radiology, you will be a PGY-2). Your intern year can be transitional, preliminary internal medicine, or surgical. While you interview for radiology programs, you must also apply and interview for these first-year programs. These first-year programs will be part of the supplemental rank order list, while your radiology programs will make up your primary rank order list. The easiest way to think about these are two separate lists; where you would like to end up for your intern year and where you would like to be for your advanced program.

Suppose you match to an advanced program (radiology) and not to a preliminary program. In that case, you must seek a first-year position during the Match Week Supplemental Offer and Acceptance Program (SOAP). If a preliminary position still needs to be attained after SOAP, the applicant is responsible for submitting to the

F. I. Chouhdry (✉)
Department of Breast Imaging, Mount Sinai Health System, Icahn School of Medicine at Mount Sinai, New York, NY, USA
e-mail: Fatima.Chouhdry@mountsinai.org

J. Shames et al. (eds.), *A Radiologist's Path*,
https://doi.org/10.1007/978-3-031-86882-5_5

NRMP a waiver of match commitment to the advanced program. Also, remember that you will only match at a preliminary position on your supplemental list if you have already matched at an advanced program.

So, how do you go about doing this? If you used the Post-it method, you probably already know where programs will fall on your rank order list. Do not try to rank programs based on your assessment of where you think you will match. The algorithm is based on your preference, trying to match you and the program at your highest pick. Only rank the programs you feel would make you happy if you matched there. The last thing you want to do is rank a program you hated and end up matching there. Try to have your rank order list submitted and certified as early as possible; you can make changes until the deadline, but better to get it done early!

Match week is the third week of March, the two most important days being Monday and Friday. On Monday, applicants will find out IF they matched. If you did match, Friday is when you find out where you matched. If you did not match, you have the rest of the week before Friday to try to find a position through SOAP. Hoping that everything goes well; you will always remember Match Week, particularly that Friday. Everyone has a Match story…the moment you find out which program will help you succeed in this next step of your career. I sincerely hope that your particular Match story is everything you desire and have worked for. Good luck!

Further Reading

National Resident Matching Program. NRMP. Accessed April 11, 2025. https://www.nrmp.org/.

Chapter 6
Transferring from a Different Specialty into Radiology

Jake A. Gibbons

Changing from one specialty to another is a major, life-altering decision. Depending on where one is in his or her career, this may require a significant investment of time and likely some degree of additional postgraduate medical training. With further training comes a probable decrease in pay and a lifestyle change. With all that being said, transitioning to a different medical specialty is a worthwhile endeavor for many physicians needing a change in their careers. Such a change has the potential to reignite the flame and restore one's passion for practicing medicine.

There are several reasons that one may choose to pursue a given specialty. Alternatively, there are often reasons that one might decide not to select another specialty. Common motivators include a genuine passion for the specialty and interest in the field with a sense of devotion toward the representative patient population. Social factors, including compensation and perceived lifestyle, are also of significant importance to many.

Traditionally, medical students spend their clinical years rotating through different specialties to identify a field for which they are most passionate. They are expected to utilize their limited experience, sometimes as little as two to four weeks, to make an informed decision regarding their field of choice. Rotations in more niche fields, such as radiology and radiation oncology, are sometimes not even included in the core curriculum at many medical schools. However, the more "popular" areas, at least from a number's standpoint, are always allocated as core rotations. These include internal medicine, general surgery, pediatrics, obstetrics & gynecology, and family medicine.

Not only are medical students lacking exposure to multiple specialties, but they are also expected to make a significant decision with often minimal experience from their clinical rotations to draw from. Sometimes, this is only a few weeks of rotating through the specialty that they ultimately apply to. Several weeks of experience in a

J. A. Gibbons (✉)
Department of Radiology, Baylor University Medical Center, Dallas, TX, USA

J. Shames et al. (eds.), *A Radiologist's Path*,
https://doi.org/10.1007/978-3-031-86882-5_6

particular field may not accurately portray what life as a physician in that field will be like. For all of these reasons, it is not unreasonable to expect that there will be medical students who end up unhappy in their chosen field at some point in their careers. For many, this realization comes as early as the internship year of residency. For others, this happens later after years of practicing in their given field.

Additionally, external factors can contribute to or necessitate a change to another specialty. This includes physical illness or disability. Priorities may change as one enters a different stage of life. What seemed exhilarating and fascinating as a medical student or resident may become exhausting later. Social pressures such as having children and raising a family are often considerations.

Historically, radiology has been regarded as an attractive specialty choice for medical graduates. The reasons for this are variable. Studies have shown that lifestyle and income are becoming increasingly important for medical students when selecting their specialty [1, 2]. Radiology, in particular, is considered to be a "lifestyle friendly" career with perceived controllable work hours and higher-than-average compensation. A study in 2005 by Newton et al. demonstrated that radiology was commonly selected as a specialty by students who heavily valued and prioritized both a favorable lifestyle and relatively high income when making their residency decision [1]. Conversely, specialties like general surgery and obstetrics & gynecology were preferentially selected by students who, on average, did not prioritize income and lifestyle [1].

Burnout is widespread among physicians in the United States. Studies suggest that approximately one in three physicians is experiencing burnout at a given time [3]. The consequences of physician burnout are vast, the most extreme of which is physician suicide. Physician suicide rates are higher than the general population [4]. The practice of clinical medicine is commonly cited as one of the primary causes of physician burnout [5]. Caring for patients is inherently stressful. There are adverse patient outcomes. Patient volumes are increasing, while compensation is declining. The burden of navigating the health insurance companies is an ever-evolving challenge of modern clinical practice. While a career in radiology by no means circumvents all of these challenges, for some, it is a perfect middle ground that quells many of the stresses of practicing clinical medicine. It is worth emphasizing, however, that burnout is also a problem in radiology, just like it is in many other fields, albeit for its own unique set of reasons. A survey of radiologists from 2022 reported that 49% of practicing radiologists were experiencing burnout [6].

Radiology is a unique field in that some or all of the radiologist's work can be performed remotely. Some radiologists even practice across state lines, reading studies performed in different parts of the country. Working remotely can promote greater lifestyle flexibility. For the procedurally inclined, radiology offers a nice mixture of procedural opportunities. Interventional radiology is an attractive option for those looking for a more heavy emphasis on procedures as part of their daily work. For those who enjoy seeing patients, subspecialties such as breast imaging and nuclear medicine allow regular patient interaction. Radiology is a broad field with many different offerings that can be uniquely tailored to fit the individual physician's needs.

Ultimately, deciding to change specialties requires much self-reflection and thought. There may be a significant psychological burden associated with such a decision. Although the outcome of changing fields might be gratifying, the stress of navigating a career change is substantial. Thoroughly exploring and weighing the risks versus benefits of switching to another field are essential steps to perform before the decision is made to make a change. Speaking extensively with loved ones and identifying mentors is worthwhile. Changing to a different medical specialty may require difficult conversations, such as with a residency program director or a partner in one's practice.

I made the decision to switch from internal medicine to radiology in my second year of internal medicine residency. As a medical student, I enjoyed both fields but ultimately decided to try clinical medicine. I also had minimal exposure to radiology as a medical student, as opposed to a three-month internal medicine clerkship. As I worked through internal medicine residency, however, I found the work less gratifying than expected. Additionally, I frequently reflected on my time as a medical student rotating through radiology, which I loved. I began spending some time in the reading rooms at my home program and enjoyed the experience. I also spoke with many of the attendings at my program, all of whom offered honest opinions about their jobs. I spoke with family and friends. I even made a pros and cons list. After much reflection, I eventually made the decision to switch. For multiple reasons unique to my situation, I decided to first finish my internal medicine training.

I spoke with my program director in internal medicine, who supported me in making the change. I explored the local radiology programs, hoping to find a vacant spot. This proved unsuccessful. So, ultimately, I decided to apply through the Electronic Residency Application Service (ERAS). I was at peace with this, as it would allow me to fully explore and interview at programs I was most interested in. Additionally, this allowed me to have a say in where I did my radiology training by making a rank list rather than moving to a different part of a country to fill a vacant residency spot. I was lucky enough to match into my first-choice radiology residency program. As I write this, I am in my first year of radiology residency and am thrilled to have made this change. I do not have any regrets and would thoroughly recommend changing specialties to anyone seriously interested in doing so.

References

1. Newton DAMD, Grayson MSMD, Thompson LF. The variable influence of lifestyle and income on medical students' career specialty choices: data from two U.S. medical schools, 1998–2004. Academic Medicine. 2005;80(9):809–14.
2. Schwartz RW, Jarecky RK, Strodel WE, Haley JV, Young B, Griffen WO. Controllable lifestyle: a new factor in career choice by medical students. Acad Med. 1989;64:606–9.
3. Shanafelt TD. Enhancing meaning in work: a prescription for preventing physician burnout and promoting patient-centered care. JAMA. 2009;302(12):1338–40.
4. Schernhammer E. Taking their own lives—the high rate of physician suicide. N Engl J Med. 2005;352(24):2473–6.
5. Drummond D. Physician burnout: its origin, symptoms, and five main causes. Fam Pract Manag. 2015;22(5):42–7.
6. Bailey CR, Bailey AM, McKenney AS, Clifford R. Understanding and appreciating burnout in radiologists. Weiss RadioGraphics. 2022;42(5):E137–9.

Chapter 7
Transferring from One Radiology Residency Program to Another

Robyn G. Roth

Transferring from One Radiology Residency Program to Another

Most people do not enter a residency program to transfer, but life happens. Speaking from experience, residents may choose to switch programs for several reasonable unforeseen circumstances, including life events, changes in health, finances, career, or even a bad fit. According to the Accreditation Council for Graduate Medical Education (ACGME), more than 1,000 residents transfer from one residency program to another each year [2] AMA.

Fortunately, there are opportunities to transfer programs if such a circumstance arises. This chapter will focus on the process and resources available if you're considering switching residency programs. I transferred radiology programs after my R1 year after meeting my husband (also a radiology resident at the time!) during my intern year, more on that later.

Things to Consider Before Transferring Programs

There are lots of legitimate unforeseen reasons why one might consider transferring programs, including but not limited to:

- Life events such as pregnancy, marriage, sickness, or death in the family
- Financial changes (loss of job of a spouse)
- Geographic concerns

R. G. Roth (✉)
Department of Radiology, Cooper University Hospital, Camden, NJ, USA
e-mail: roth-robyn@CooperHealth.edu

© The Author(s), under exclusive license to Springer Nature Switzerland AG 2025
J. Shames et al. (eds.), *A Radiologist's Path*,
https://doi.org/10.1007/978-3-031-86882-5_7

- Change in career (switching to another specialty or leaving medicine altogether)
- *Possibly even a lousy fit* * (proceed with caution with this reason)

It is important to remember that transferring programs may have a significant impact on your personal and professional relationships if not executed properly, so it's in your best interest to have a legitimate reason for wanting to transfer programs (no—seeking a higher academic status does not qualify as a good excuse).

If you are considering transferring programs, inform your program director immediately. You will ultimately need their support to transfer programs successfully, so it's best to be transparent from the start. Most program directors will understand and support your decision as long as you have a legitimate reason. They may even be willing to work with you to find a mutually beneficial situation. Full transparency will serve you in the long run (i.e., don't go behind their back!).

Though transfers can occur at any time during the academic year, most tend to occur on July 1. That said, residencies may have unexpected openings at any time throughout the year, so it's best to be prepared if an opportunity presents itself. Transferring programs can take a few months to prepare your application and identify a program successfully, so begin the process as soon as you know the situation.

Some wisdom to all residents: **job interviews begin on day one of residency.** Be a stellar resident regardless of your intention to stay or transfer. No matter your circumstance, you will likely need letters of recommendation from your current attendings and will likely cross paths with former residents and attendings in the future. The radiology world is small, so be careful not to burn bridges on your way out. Also, there is no guarantee that you will be able to transfer programs, so it is essential to maintain a good relationship with your current program, no matter the outcome.

Steps to Transferring Radiology Residencies

1. **Research.** If you hope to transfer residencies, scour the resources listed below to find potential openings. Become active in message boards trying to identify a swap or transfer. Reach out to friends at other programs. Trust me—some prestigious programs may not advertise an opening not to jeopardize their reputation.
2. **Prepare.** Early in the process, write a general email template to programs with potential openings, including your name, current program, reasons for transferring, and what you could bring to the program. Be clear and concise. Attach your CV, letters of recommendation, and even a letter of good standing from your program.
3. **Openly communicate with your program (i.e., do not try to transfer programs behind their back).** Transparency is key! As mentioned, inform your program director immediately if you are considering transferring programs. You

will ultimately need their support to transfer programs successfully, so it's best to be transparent from the start. Going behind their back may have significant personal and professional consequences. Most program directors will understand and support your decision as long as you have a legitimate reason; they may even be willing to work with you to find a mutually beneficial situation. Since there is no guarantee that you will be able to transfer programs, it is essential to maintain a good relationship with your current program, no matter the outcome.

4. **Obtain letters of recommendation and a letter of good standing from your current program.** Once you make your intentions about transferring known, start asking for letters of recommendation from attendings in your current program. You will also ultimately need a letter of good standing from your program director, so it is essential to maintain a professional relationship throughout the transferring process. **Reach out to other programs and residents.** Send out your email template, including your CV, letters of recommendation, and reasons for transferring to any openings that might be a good fit. Consider emailing program directors of desirable residencies even if there is no official opening. Unexpected openings always happen, so they may keep your information on file if such a circumstance arises. Also, take into account the power of networking. Reach out to any residents and attendings you know at other programs to inquire about potential openings. Networking with others is often the best way to find coveted spots before they are advertised (prestigious programs may not announce an opening for fear of damaging their reputation). In an ideal world, you can find a resident at another program who wants to **swap,** described in detail below, which may be mutually beneficial for both programs. If you're happy with your training location but wish to switch specialties, consider reaching out to the program director at your current institution, which may make for a smoother transition.

Transferring Versus Swapping

Transferring is the process of switching from one residency to another leaving your former program down a resident, which may negatively impact your program and department. On the other hand, **swapping** indicates a mutual transfer where two equivalent residents at different programs choose to switch spots. Swapping is usually a better situation for both programs since no one loses a resident, but executing a successful swap can be complicated. Most successful swaps occur through networking and word of mouth. Therefore, most switches are transfers rather than swaps.

Resources for Residents Interested in Swapping/Vacating Residency Spots [3] (Grisham)

Student Doctor Network (SDN) – an online forum for medical students, residents, and attendings. Keep your eyes open for openings that may not be advertised! It's also a great way to connect with other residents looking to transfer, potentially swapping programs (*https://www.studentdoctor.net*).

ResidencySwap – an online organization that helps residents fill vacant residency spots or swap spots with other residents. Allows anonymous posts of people looking to swap residencies and notifies you of any openings. It also offers a "Together Anywhere" mode designed for couples looking for programs in geographical proximity to each other.

    Cost: $60 a month (*https://www.residentswap.org/*).

FREIDA, the AMA Residency and Fellowship Database – allows you to search for a residency or fellowship from more than 12,000 programs, all accredited by the Accreditation Council for Graduate Medical Education (ACGME), free for AMA members (Students, $20/year | Residents, $45/year).

FindAResident – the AAMC's online service to connect program directors and residents. Programs share information about openings and applicants post resumes for programs to review. Most vacancies open at the beginning of the year, in December and late March. Cost: $75 feed for applicants or $30 fee for active ERAS users (*https://systems.aamc.org/findaresident/*).

MedResidency – a website that allows you to search for specialty, geographic location, and training level. Cost: $39 a month (*https://medresidency.com/*).

Unmatched MD – similar to above. Cost: $45 a month (*https://unmatchedmd.com*).

Facebook Groups, Twitter, and Social Media – do not underestimate the power of social media. Check radiology-specific Facebook groups (i.e., Radiology Chicks) frequently for unexpected openings, and consider posting anonymously with what you are looking for. Interact with other radiology residents, attendings, and program directors on X and verbalize (publicly or through private messages) your desire to transfer programs. Follow other residency programs on Instagram/X, which may also post unexpected openings.

Network – networking is essential for anyone looking to transfer. Connect with former co-interns, medical students, mentors, and friends who may have insider information about other programs and can help advocate on your behalf. Attend medical conferences, making a point to connect with residents and attendings at other programs. Make your intentions known.

Swapping If Your Residency Is Closing

Unfortunately, residency programs can close, leaving displaced residents scrambling for openings elsewhere. Thankfully, transferring in this situation is more accessible because your funding will follow you to your new program. The ACGME will allow the other program to exceed its normal residency cap in these special circumstances.

My Personal Experience Transferring Radiology Residencies

I attended medical school at Albert Einstein College of Medicine in the Bronx, NY. On Match Day 2008, I was ecstatic when I received my top choices for internship (a transitional year at Albert Einstein Hospital in Philadelphia, PA) and radiology residency at my home institution, Montefiore Hospital in New York.

I planned on staying in Philadelphia for precisely one year to take a break from the hustle and bustle of New York, but life had other plans. During my intern year in Philadelphia, I met my future husband, who was also matched into a radiology residency in the area. We dated throughout our internship, but our year together ended when I moved back to NY in July to begin my radiology residency. Though we dated long distance, it soon became apparent that this was the man I would marry.

As a couple, we decided that he would pursue transferring to a NY program, mainly because there were more programs and more potential spots. He informed his program director early in the year about his intention to transfer, who was supportive. Despite his efforts, he was unsuccessful finding a suitable radiology opening. As the academic year approached, we all but gave up and planned to move midway to commute to our respective programs.

In May of my R1 year (i.e., almost the end of the academic year), I received an unsolicited text from a friend from my intern year living in Philadelphia. "Did you hear there is a radiology opening at the Hospital of the University of Pennsylvania?" I had not. This was not an advertised position; I was only alerted through word of mouth.

Indeed, this was too good to be true; I hadn't even received an interview from Penn during my initial Match application. I ran home and frantically gathered my CV. I wrote a heartfelt email to the program director about my situation and stared at my computer all night until I received a response. She responded hours later, requesting my in-service scores (yikes!) and a reference, which I happily provided. She called me later that day, asking me to come to an interview. I sat down with my program director and informed him that an unexpected opening at Penn had essentially fallen in my lap, and I had to pursue it. His response was, "love is love!"

I interviewed at Penn the next day, and they offered me the position on the train ride home. I unapologetically accepted. As ecstatic as I was, I did experience some negativity from my former residents, mainly because they lost a resident in the call pool. Still, those negative feelings subsided as the years went by, and I ultimately had to do what was best for myself and my future family.

I finished my R1 year at Montefiore and started at Penn on July 1, where I completed my residency and fellowship. I married my husband later that year, and we settled down in the Philadelphia area with our three young children.

My transfer experience is far from typical, but it highlights the importance of networking and much luck during the process.

Advice to Anyone Considering Transferring Programs

Successfully transferring programs requires patience, networking, and much luck. Keep going, especially if making the transfer is important to you. If you are unsuccessful at transferring programs, try to improve your current situation and learn from your experience. Note what was not a good fit so you do not make the same mistake in the future. Remember that residency is a temporary position and will likely be done in around 4/5 years, after which you can easily change paths.

Best of luck wherever your path takes you.

Tips for Anyone Considering Transferring Programs
Be transparent and have a legitimate reason for wanting to transfer. Most program directors will be supportive of your decision and may even be willing to work with you to find a mutually beneficial situation.

Prepare your application including an email template with the reason for wanting to transfer, CV, and letters of recommendation; unexpected openings can become available at any time throughout the academic year.

Utilize the resources described above, but do not underestimate the power of networking.

Be a stellar resident, no matter your circumstance. The radiology world is small, and job interviews begin on day one.

References

1. Carter, Crystal. Residency Programs: Why and How to Transfer. https://www.practicematch.com/physicians/articles/residencyprograms-why-and-how-to-transfer.cfm. Accessed April 3 2025..
2. Grisham EMD. A guide to swapping residency programs. https://elitemedicalprep.com/a-guide-to-swapping-residencyprograms/. Accessed 27 Feb 2023..
3. Want to switch residency programs? Five things you should know. AMA Staff Writer. https://www.ama-assn.org/medicalresidents/residency-life/want-switch-residecency. Accessed 27 Feb 2023..

Chapter 8
Radiology Residency and the International Medical Graduate (IMG)

Rashmi Balasubramanya

Radiology is a sought-after specialty for an international medical graduate (IMG) coming to the United States. At the same time, some of the global medical graduates are US citizens (US IMGs); a more significant proportion are not US citizens but are international medical graduates (non-US IMGs).

Radiology Residency for the International Medical Graduate

The number of IMGs matching into diagnostic radiology residency programs has progressively increased. The proportion of non-US IMGs in diagnostic radiology residencies rose from 4.4% in 2006 to 9.4% in 2020 [1]. While part of this is due to the increase in residency spots, IMGs also come with unique advantages, such as completing a residency in their home country and consequently having an increased number of presentations and publications at the time of the match. This group brings diverse experience to the applicant pool. The decline in US medical graduates applying to diagnostic radiology helped propel these numbers. Some non-US IMGs prefer the diagnostic residency pathway to the alternate path due to the uncertainties of the alternate route at times.

R. Balasubramanya (✉)
Department of Radiology, Thomas Jefferson University Hospital, Philadelphia, PA, USA
e-mail: Rashmi.balasubramanya@jefferson.edu

© The Author(s), under exclusive license to Springer Nature   41
Switzerland AG 2025
J. Shames et al. (eds.), *A Radiologist's Path*,
https://doi.org/10.1007/978-3-031-86882-5_8

USMLE Score

To be a highly competitive residency candidate, high USMLE scores are a prerequisite to obtaining a diagnostic radiology residency. The mean Step 2 USMLE score for the non-US IMG who matched into diagnostic radiology in 2022 through the NRMP match process was 250 [2], and the unmatched non-US IMG was 245, which highlights the highly competitive nature of this pool of applicants.

Publications

The mean number of publications for non-US IMG who matched in radiology for the year 2022 was 16.9 as compared to 7 for the matched US-IMG [3]. This also shows the highly qualified nature of this group of candidates.

US Letters of Recommendation

Though this group is highly qualified, a US letter of recommendation is invariably required to increase the chances of matching into a diagnostic radiology residency. Part of this is because residency program directors may not be acquainted with non-US faculty and institutions. In addition, most letter writers outside the United States may need to familiarize themselves with the requisites of a US residency letter of recommendation. Working in the US health system to get a letter of recommendation also provides the non-US IMG the opportunity to understand the nuances before joining a residency.

Research Experience

Procuring research positions bolsters the chance of matching in a radiology residency. For applicants with a weaker resume, this research not only allows for publications and presentations to enhance your application but also allows you to secure strong letters of recommendation. An efficient way to increase visibility is presenting papers and attending the yearly Radiological Society of North America (RSNA) conferences. This also allows the opportunity to network with other program directors and mentors.

Social media is a new tool to increase the visibility of applicants. Following residency programs on Twitter and Instagram, highlighting and commenting about cases and papers is a way for applicants to "get themselves out there" [4].

Alternate Pathway

Radiology is one of the few specialties which allows the alternate pathway. Radiologists who have completed a diagnostic radiology residency in countries other than the United States and Canada and want to practice in the United States can follow the international medical graduates alternate pathway. Instead of a traditional residency followed by a fellowship, these candidates can become board eligible by working four years, as fellows or attendings in different subdivisions of radiology, at one institution within eight years of graduation. The by-product is that this group is immensely qualified, as this supersedes their previous training in radiology.

Visa Status

For a non-US IMG who wants to practice in the United States, procuring a US visa is paramount as the residency, fellowship, and subsequent practice as an attending depends on the visa type. US-IMGs are invariably green card holders or citizens, making the pathway much easier. Not all visas are created equal. Some are more valuable than others, while some are easier to obtain. Below are the most commonly used visas.

H1B Visa

This is a dual-intent visa for temporary workers who hold professional degrees. H1B allows the physician to be employed in the United States for up to six years. All physicians qualify for the basic requirements of an H1B visa, as being a physician is a specialty occupation. ECFMG certification and a state medical license are other requirements for obtaining an H1B visa. Most hospitals are nonprofit organizations without the H1B visa cap, which applies to other H1B applicants. Large university hospitals tend to sponsor J1 visas, and smaller community hospitals with residency programs sponsor H1B visas. Generally, the trend has been to sponsor J1 visas, not H1B visas.

The six-year period is sufficient to cover a five-year radiology residency and one year of fellowship but, immediately after, requires the applicant to procure another visa or a green card. Options at this stage would include applying for a green card or O1 visa.

O1 Visa   for Individuals with Extraordinary Ability or Achievement.

This highly sought-after visa has benefits over the H1B visa as there is no time limit, and it can be extended indefinitely. However, the criteria for obtaining an O1 visa are stringent [5], like the EB1 category green card. In short, this requires the applicant to have published extensively. As a note, it would make better sense for radiologists in training to publish extensively to be eligible for this visa later.

J1 Visa

This accounts for the most common visa for non-US IMGs. The J1 visa is an exchange visitor visa sponsored by the ECFMG. In addition to having a valid ECFMG certificate, this visa requires a Statement of Need from the country of last permanent residence, which states the need for specialized training for the applicant. The major disadvantage of a J1 visa is that the physician should return to their home country for two years after completing the residency. Another downside is that the J1 visa typically needs renewal every year. Upon completion of training, the J1 visa holders must return to their home country for two years or receive a waiver, which commonly requires the applicant to work in an underserved community [6]. Other options include working in the Department of VA (Veterans Affairs). The waiver also requires the applicant to establish that the applicant's spouse and children would face exceptional hardship should the applicant leave the United States for two years. One advantage of working in underserved communities is that it offers tremendous financial benefits. Upon completing the waiver, the radiologist can take another step toward becoming a US citizen by converting to an H1B or O1 visa or applying for a green card.

Green Card

It is said that the path of progress could be smoother. Similarly, most IMGs have an uphill battle completing the residency and fellowship and maintaining their visa. Most radiologists who come to the United States for a residency program want to become US citizens; a green card is the second step after obtaining a visa.

Green cards come in assorted flavors, but for a physician, employment-based green cards such as EB1 (Extraordinary Ability) [7] or EB2 (National Interest Waiver –NIW) [8] categories are most applicable.

EB1 Category Green Cards

This particular category of green cards for physicians and scientists can be equated to the royal path. It has stringent criteria to prove that one is indeed extraordinary. For physicians, this means having extensive publications, including multiple first-author publications and plenty of citations for these publications. Being a reviewer for major medical journals also satisfies some requirements for this category of green card. It helps to show that the physician plays a leading or critical role in an organization and commands a high salary compared to others in the same field. National or internationally recognized awards help prove the physician is of extraordinary caliber. This category of green cards is beneficial for radiologists from countries like India and China who cannot obtain an EB2 category green card as there is a wait time of 10 years or more due to the yearly quota of EB2 green cards issued for a country regardless of the population size [9].

The prudent radiologist should start publishing extensively and take up leadership roles during residency, keeping this requirement in mind. It would also help to be in an academic practice instead of private practice upon completion of residency as obtaining EB1 category green card is more accessible in an educational setting. The EB1b (outstanding professor or researcher) subtype of EB1 category green cards requires evidence of only two of the eight requisites and establishing that the applicant is involved in high-end research [7]. This also means showing that the radiologist is working in a university setting.

The EB1A subtype requires establishing evidence for three of the eight criteria and is more stringent but can be self-petitioned.

EB2 or (National Interest Waiver) NIW Category Green Card

This is a self-petition green card. One subtype requires the applicant to work in an underserved area or at the veterans administration institution for at least five years. Another subtype involves the establishment of exceptional ability **and** that the United States would benefit by allowing the applicant to live in the United States permanently. The US national interest can be established by providing evidence that the presence of the physician/radiologist in the United States would improve the health of Americans or the US economy. The requirements of the EB2 category are more accessible to fulfill than the EB1A category. They are a good route for most non-US IMGs except radiologists from countries like India and China. The employment category green card for these two countries has a long backlog of at least ten years.

It would help international medical graduates know this long timeline and brace themselves by publishing extensively during residency. Some useful websites are provided. The following are useful websites for IMGs applying to diagnostic radiology residency:

1. https://www.ama-assn.org/education/international-medical-education
2. https://www.uscis.gov
3. https://www.nrmp.org/match-data-analytics/residency-data-reports
4. https://www.theabr.org/diagnostic-radiology/initial-certification/alternative-pathways

References

1. https://www.nrmp.org/wp-content/uploads/2022/05/2022-Main-Match-Results-and-Data_Final.pdf
2. https://www.nrmp.org/match-data-analytics/residency-data-reports/
3. https://www.nrmp.org/wp-content/uploads/2022/07/Charting-Outcomes-IMG-2022_Final.pdf
4. Czawlytko C, Smith E, Awan O, Resnik C, Hossain R. The effect of virtual interviews and social media on applicant decision-making during the 2020-2021 resident match cycle. Acad Radiol. 2022;29(6):928–34.
5. https://www.uscis.gov/working-in-the-united-states/temporary-workers/o-1-visa-individuals-with-extraordinary-ability-or-achievement
6. https://www.ama-assn.org/education/international-medical-education/immigration-information-international-medical-graduates
7. https://www.uscis.gov/working-in-the-united-states/permanent-workers/employment-based-immigration-first-preference-eb-1
8. https://www.uscis.gov/working-in-the-united-states/permanent-workers/employment-based-immigration-second-preference-eb-2
9. https://www.statista.com/chart/16528/long-wait-times-for-green-cards/

Chapter 9
Abdominal Fellowship

Anne Kathryn Misiura

Introduction

So, you've decided you want to take on the pancreas? Cheers, my friend. It is not for the weak. Abdominal imaging is challenging, time-consuming, and undeniably rewarding. At the end of one year, you'll be amazed at how much you've seen and done, and you'll look forward to the future landscape of advanced body imaging.

Body, or abdominal imaging, is a tough nugget of a subspecialty that can be further divided and subspecialized as you fine-tune your interests. You may plan on an academic career and see yourself leading hepatocellular carcinoma tumor boards biweekly. Perhaps, you're headed to a private practice or community radiology position and will one day be the GI and GU guru your referring docs call for their most complex cases. Either way, you've chosen a wise area of expertise and you'll always be in great demand. Let's talk about how you'll get there.

Application Process

Abdominal/body imaging fellowships are not in the Match. In the past years, this resulted in a less-than-ideal situation of rolling admissions, no structured national timeframe, and a "free for all" experience for candidates. It was not unheard of for residents in their second year to begin courting abdominal fellowship programs before being fully exposed to the field of radiology. Most fortunately, as a result of the Society of Chairs of Academic Radiology Departments (SCARD) policy statement in 2010, since the 2021-2022 cycle, there is now a structured timeline to

A. K. Misiura (✉)
Department of Radiology, Thomas Jefferson University Hospital, Philadelphia, PA, USA
e-mail: anne.misiura@jefferson.edu

J. Shames et al. (eds.), *A Radiologist's Path*,
https://doi.org/10.1007/978-3-031-86882-5_9

pursuing an abdominal fellowship, and most programs have opted into this collegial process of interviewing. Most programs begin the application process during the fall of your R3 year (i.e. Fall 2024 application process begins for the 2026-2027 position). You should check with individual programs to confirm their deadlines.

Unlike the residency application process or other fellowships in the Match, you're in the driver's seat to move at your speed, look for directions, and make your own decisions toward your final destination. Arguably, this process is a bit more work at the beginning to collect information on potential programs and individually complete required applications—but in the end, you've accepted a position before your co-residents in other subspecialties.

If you haven't already, now is the time to get familiar with the Society of Abdominal Radiology (and join if you haven't! Membership fees are waived for members-in-training). They have an excellent database for fellowship programs organized by state/region to get you started on your search [1]. As of this publication, they only list programs that have opted into the collegial SCARD guidelines recruitment process. These programs have agreed to a standardized timeline as outlined in Table 9.1. If you are interested in and applying to a program outside of this process, pay special attention to their specific deadlines.

The application packet is pretty standard across the board, but keeping a spreadsheet of the required documents for each program would behoove you to ensure you don't forget something. You are responsible for individually submitting your packets and providing their delivery. Many programs have electronic applications, at least in part, but it's still on you to gather the required documents to upload. Most of the usual requirements are listed in Table 9.2. Get it done in a timely fashion.

More often than not, the last piece of the application will be waiting for your letters of recommendation from the writers. Ask early, and remind gently and constantly.

Now is an excellent time to get some passport photos taken. If you don't use them now, you'll probably use them in the next 5 years for credentialing or renewing that passport.

Table 9.1 Standardized timeline

November 1st, 2024: First day applications can be accepted
January 13th, 2025 - March 31st, 2025: Interview period
January 27th, 2025 Noon standard time: No fellowship may offer acceptances before this time
Applicants have until noon eastern standard time on January 29th to accept or decline any offer made BEFORE January 29th. For any offer made ON or AFTER January 29th, the candidate has a 1 day grace period (noon eastern standard time) to accept or decline the offer.

Table 9.2 List of requirements	Individual institution application
	CV with no gaps in the timeline after medical school using standard date/year format
	Personal statement
	Copy of your USMLE (steps 1–3) or COMLEX scores
	Medical school transcript
	Medical school dean's letter
	Letter of good standing from the program director
	Two to three additional letters of recommendation
	Photograph (some may require passport-quality photos for standardization)

What to Look for in a Program

Not all programs are created equally. Of course, every program will likely have you spend time in ultrasound, CT, and MRI, but the mileage may vary, and additional rotations in light biopsy service, nuclear medicine, advanced applications, and other electives are routinely offered. Take advantage of these options. A great program will work with you to craft a schedule to help you prepare for your first job. When you apply, I wager that most of you have no idea what kind of position you'll accept your first year out of training. But most of you will sign contracts for your first job during fellowship, if not the year before, as in the current market. If you've accepted a position where you'll be expected to read PET scans and perform thyroid biopsies or hysterosalpingograms, improving these skills in fellowship would be great.

The Interview

Schedule interviews as early as you can. The early bird gets the worm. Programs following the SCARD guidelines can start sending out offers as soon as the first interview day, so if you have a number one dream fellowship spot, be there that first week.

There is no abdominal fellowship-specific advice for interviewing. You've done this dozens of times already at this point in your life, though maybe it's your first time dealing with virtual interviews. As of February 2023, abdominal fellowship interviews are still being conducted virtually. The same basic interview principles apply, though you'll need to spend some prep time setting up your interview space and securing your internet connection. There are endless resources online for thriving in a virtual interview, and it wouldn't hurt to spend an evening glancing over some of these.

Be thoughtful. Dress professionally. Prepare your interview space. This is your time to ask questions, so have them (bonus to virtual interviews is that you can have questions written down right in front of you, but please don't make it seem like you're reading a script). Your application packet and references speak for your abilities, but the interview is what makes you an individual. Interviewers want to ensure you're personable, so show them who you are. And relax.

Take advantage of any opportunity to speak with current fellows. I learned the most about my fellowship during the casual lunch with a current fellow. If you cannot be there in person, ask for the contact information of the current fellows and send them some open-ended questions about the program.

Take 2 min after each interview to write down your initial thoughts, what you talked about, follow-up questions, and anything else. It's not expected, but it certainly doesn't hurt to send a quick note to your interviewers thanking them for their time. Keep it brief. Mention something you enjoyed discussing. This shows them you're interested!

Accepting a Position

Here's where your debriefing notes come in. Hopefully, you have some gut feelings about where you'd like to end up. With the current SCARD guidelines, you'll hopefully begin receiving offers right after your interview. If that offer comes between January 27th and 28th, you have until January 29th at noon to accept that offer. After that, rolling admissions come back to play, and programs only give you 24 hours to accept or reject an offer. This is why it behooves you to schedule early and prioritize interviews at your most preferred institutions.

But don't worry, not all programs fill up in January. Don't fret if you didn't get your dream spot or you're late to the game. Watch program websites and social media for late open positions outside this cycle. Life happens. It'll work out how it's supposed to.

Welcome to abdominal imaging! I'm biased, but I think we're fantastic.

Reference

1. SAR Fellowships Map. Society of Abdominal Radiology. [cited 2023Feb25]. Available from: https://abdominalradiology.org/sar-fellowships-map/

Chapter 10
Breast Imaging Fellowship

Suzanne McElligott and Ekta Gupta

Breast Imaging as a Subspecialty Field

Breast cancer is the most frequently diagnosed cancer and the leading cause of cancer-related death in women [1]. Mammographic screening has been proven to reduce morbidity and mortality from breast cancer [2, 3]. Multimodality breast imaging can increase the diagnostic accuracy of nonpalpable breast lesions [1]. Several studies have found that multidisciplinary collaboration for breast cancer patients has improved care [4].

Breast imaging is an essential subspecialty in radiology. It plays a crucial role in breast cancer diagnosis and treatment planning. Within this discipline, breast imaging practice has been regulated and standardized. In 1997, the US Food and Drug Administration published guidelines for implementing the Mammography Quality Standards Act (MQSA), including requirements for physicians interpreting mammography. Most of these requirements became effective in 1999 [5].

As the demand for mammography and other breast imaging studies increases with an aging population and increased compliance with mammographic recommendations, there is also increased demand for mammogram interpretation to be performed by radiologists with subspecialty training in breast imaging [6].

S. McElligott (✉) · E. Gupta
Department of Radiology, Zucker School of Medicine at Hofstra Northwell Health,
Lake Success, NY, USA
e-mail: smcellig@northwell.edu; egupta@northwell.edu

© The Author(s), under exclusive license to Springer Nature
Switzerland AG 2025
J. Shames et al. (eds.), *A Radiologist's Path*,
https://doi.org/10.1007/978-3-031-86882-5_10

Why Should I Choose or Not Choose This Field?

Historically, many radiologists learned their breast imaging skills on the job when they were responsible for reading mammograms within their practices. Study data suggest that fellowship-trained and experienced breast imagers have patients and healthcare plans increasingly seeking improved accuracy and subspecialty training [7]. As the need for breast imagers continues to increase, with higher demand than workforce supply, ongoing job opportunities are projected. One study in the United States in 2009 predicted that the small number of graduating radiologists that enter the field of breast imaging would result in a reduced breast imaging workforce over the subsequent 15–20 years [8].

In addition to job opportunities, a 2008 survey cited other advantages of a career in breast imaging, including a flexible work schedule and few calls or emergencies [7]. Breast imaging is primarily an outpatient practice which can be appealing to some residents after spending years of training within a hospital setting, handling countless medical emergencies.

There are additional considerations for residents before they commit to the field. Breast imaging is one of the subspecialties in radiology that offers the most patient interaction. Direct patient contact makes breast imaging a challenging but rewarding subspecialty. Breast radiologists take ownership of patient care by having the ability to recall patients, diagnose cancer, often be the first to convey a cancer diagnosis, play an active role in multidisciplinary rounds for the management of breast cancer patients, and subsequently follow up patients post-op as they return for their routine imaging.

Comprehensive training in breast imaging requires competency in breast interventional procedures. Although the option exists to choose a job after training that does not involve performing procedures, the procedural aspect of the subspecialty is particularly appealing to some trainees. It is a critical component of fellowship training.

In breast imaging practice, there are many pathologic diagnoses you will be responsible for knowing about and managing. However, these are predominantly breast specific, which likely appeals to some but not all radiologists as they consider career options. Breast imaging patients will be primarily adult females, and breast imagers (81%, according to a 2021 article by Haken et al.) are more likely to be female than in other radiology subspecialties [9].

Surveys conducted in 2008 and 2011 citing trainees' perceptions about why not to enter breast imaging as a subspeciality career choice include large workload, high stress, low reimbursement, and high malpractice risk [6, 7]. As a breast imager, you will multitask with your day, including a combination of procedures, reading imaging studies, following up with surgeons and patients about pathology results and management, and teaching trainees. However, following training, breast imagers can seek out flexible schedules and even fully remote work that involves reading a combination of screening and, diagnostic mammography, and breast MRI studies. Practice can involve a high percentage of breast interventional procedures or none.

What Is the Training for a Breast Imager?

Historically, it was common for radiologists reading mammography in a practice group to receive on-the-job training. For the reasons mentioned previously, this has become less common [6, 7]. Increasingly, residents practicing breast imaging are expected to have subspecialty training [10].

Breast imaging fellowships are not accredited through the Accreditation Council for Graduate Medical Education (ACGME). As a result, fellowship training can vary from one program to another. However, there are established guidelines that help standardize breast fellows' training.

In 2021, The American College of Radiology/Society of Breast Imaging published an updated fellowship training guide in the Journal of Breast Imaging: The American College of Radiology/Society of Breast Imaging Updated Fellowship Training Curriculum for Breast Imaging. They reported that they aimed to develop well-rounded fellowship graduates who could become breast imaging leaders within their practices [11, 12].

The current curriculum focuses on four main components of fellowship training, outlined in detail in the updated guidelines by Katzen, available as a link on the SBI website. Trainees should familiarize themselves with this curriculum to identify programs that will offer adequate training to attain these skills during their fellowship year. The four discrete skill sets of the training curriculum are: [11]

1. Clinical factors.
2. Noninterpretative factors.
3. Collaborative factors.
4. Scholarly factors.

Within the clinical training component, fellows must demonstrate proficiency in performing all breast imaging procedures, including biopsies and localizations using mammography, ultrasound, stereotactic/tomosynthesis, and MRI guidance [11, 12]. Trainees should inquire about the types and number of procedures they can perform during their training.

Additionally, there is a focus on noninterpretive skills. These encompass knowledge of the practice audit, quality control, risk assessment models, MRI artifacts, and safety and patient interaction. Multidisciplinary care is also emphasized. Scholarly activities include opportunities for teaching, dedicated fellow lecture series, and opportunities to attend local and national meetings [11].

Trainees must comply with all MQSA requirements for practice. All interpreting physicians must have documentation that they have met the following minimum MQSA-required qualifications listed on the MQSA website and in the ACR Practice Parameter for performing screening and diagnostic mammography [13].

How Much Time Is Enough for a Full-Year Dedicated Breast Imaging Fellowship Versus a Part-Year/Combined Fellowship?

Presently, the SBI promotes a minimum of 9 months of dedicated training in breast imaging for a fellowship year. However, it does accept programs that offer between 6 and 12 months of full-time training after residency [12, 14].

Combined programs used to be more common but have been replaced to a large extent by programs with 12 months of training in breast imaging. Breast imaging now has more diagnostic and procedural modalities to learn, and there is a new emphasis on the nonclinical competencies outlined in the ACR/SBI updated curriculum. In a survey of programs offering breast imaging published in 2014 by Farria, for the 2014–2015 academic year, 78% of the fellowships provided 9–12 months of training, and 22% provided 6 months [7]. More recent data from 2020 notes that out of 90 fellowships that participated in the Match, 84% provided 12 months of breast imaging training, and 15–16% were women's imaging or combined fellowships, usually breast/body fellowships [15].

Application Process

A fellowship called Match for Breast Imaging was established in 2017 and sponsored by the Society of Breast Imaging. According to the SBI, the fellowship Match aims to improve the interviewing process and offer resident positions. To be eligible for the Match, programs must be accredited or affiliated with an ACGME program. They must agree to the rules and timeline the National Resident Matching Program sets [16].

The SBI encourages programs offering 6 months or more in breast imaging to participate in the Match. The SBI presently lists over 70 institutions offering one or more training programs with at least 6 months of breast imaging training on their website as participating in the Match for the training year commencing in July 2024 [12].

There are also training programs that are outside the Match. Identifying these programs can be more difficult since they are not compiled in a registry on the SBI website like the Match participating programs are. For out-of-Match positions, you must rely on word of mouth, social media, review of individual institute websites, and direct contact with a program's representative for specifics about the training program, including application requirements and deadlines. As with programs that do participate in the Match, these programs can combine training in breast imaging with training in other subspecialties, including but not limited to women's imaging and body imaging.

If you are considering a combined training program, we strongly encourage you to speak with as many people as possible about the pros and cons of doing so. This is often a decision based upon personal factors, including interests and specific goals or job prospects after training.

Applying to a Breast Imaging Fellowship Through the Match

The SBI and NRMP websites provide comprehensive guidance on applying to fellowship programs through the Match, with contact information also provided for questions you may have along the way.

The timeline for each year's NRMP Match is posted on both the SBI and NRMP websites at the beginning of each academic year.

For the 2023 Radiology Breast Imaging Fellowship Match for 2024 appointments, the timeline is listed below: [12]

- August 1, 2022: Programs may accept applications.
- November 7, 2022: Virtual interview period begins.
- March 22, 2023: Match opens.
- March 31, 2023: Last day of the interview period.
- April 19, 2023: The ranking period opens.
- May 31, 2023: The ranking period closes.
- June 14, 2023: Match Day.
- July 1, 2024: Training commences.

Both websites provide more details related to the process, and the SBI website provides a Fellowship Match Universal Application, required by all participating programs and many programs that join out of the Match. The website also offers many helpful tips and answers to common questions. If you plan to apply for a breast imaging position, you should familiarize yourself with these websites and the resources for prospective candidates.

Applying

Applicants apply for fellowships 2 years before their anticipated start date. Since programs may begin accepting applications in the summer, reviewing the SBI universal application and Match program-specific requirements is a good idea beforehand. Applicants will need letters of recommendation for their applications (three required). They should allow time for the submitters to write these and choose people who can write strong letters on their behalf. Applicants should gather necessary application materials, revise their CVs, and write their personal statements early to be ready when the Match system opens for applications. Once programs have reviewed applications, they will begin offering interviews. The Match timeline will allow you to see the opening day for applications.

Spend time on your personal statement. A personal statement should be used to set you apart from other applicants. From our experience, fellowship program directors read these and value the unique insights they offer about a candidate's decision to enter the field. Please make sure they are well-written and free of grammar and spelling mistakes.

In preparing for the interview, read "SBI Tips for Residents: What Program Directors Look for in Desirable Candidates." Learn about the programs that you are applying to and be prepared to answer questions such as why you chose breast imaging and why you would choose a particular program.

Other things applicants can do to present themselves as strong applicants include involvement in breast imaging-related projects and joining the Society of Breast Imaging (SBI). SBI offers free membership to trainees to gain access to training materials that include the newsletter and opportunities for networking and making research contacts, as well as access to a career center with current job listings, including open fellowship positions.

We have yet to determine how many programs you should apply to. Historically, breast imaging fellowship has not been among the most competitive radiology fellowships; however, its popularity has increased [17, 18]. Presently, more breast imaging positions are available than applicants, with some programs more competitive than others based on their reputation or location.

Fellowship Match Summary 2018 Appointments [17]

Number of applicants—124.
Number of positions—148 filled—78.4%.
Unfilled position—24.

Fellowship Match Summary 2022 Appointments [18]

Number of applicants—141.
Number of positions—169 filled—78.15%.
Unfilled position—28.

Since 2019, there has been a shift from in-person to virtual interviews due to COVID. Unlike the radiology residency Match, which has seen an increased number of applications to each program under the virtual platform, the same has not been shown for breast fellowship applications. In a recent survey by Mullen, breast imaging fellowship program directors did not find a significant increase in the number of applications received or the number of applicants interviewed when comparing in-person interviews in 2019 and virtual interviews in 2020 [19]. They found that in 2019, 22% of applicants applied to greater than 15 programs while the rest applied to fewer. In 2020, 35% of applicants applied to greater than 15 programs [19].

What to Look For in a Program and How to Make the Most of Your Fellowship Year

Be familiar with the SBI breast imaging fellowship curriculum and look for programs that will prepare you to meet all the requirements to become a competent breast imager who can successfully practice in a clinical or academic setting and be able to provide the best care.

Choose a program with a culture that you believe you can thrive in. Look for a program that offers the opportunity for mentors and sponsors. These individuals can help to provide a head start toward a successful and rewarding career. During training, establish connections with the multidisciplinary care team, including the breast surgeon, pathologists, oncologists, radiation oncologists, and other team members participating in patient care. They can be valuable sources of information concerning understanding patient management and helpful contacts for your future career. Seek opportunities to be part of projects that interest you and that you can learn from. Instruct the medical students and residents you have contact with. Teaching is an excellent way to reinforce your knowledge, and it can help identify gaps in your knowledge base. And remember, the residents and medical students are your future colleagues.

Breast imaging, like radiology in general, involves substantial self-directed learning. Read as much as you can! Read about every new pathology, procedure, and treatment that you encounter during your training.

And most importantly, enjoy your training year. Fellows have the fantastic opportunity to specialize in the area of radiology they are passionate about. There will be attendings with years of individual and cumulative experience and wisdom to guide you, and you will have the opportunity to make meaningful connections with patients and the entire breast imaging staff at your training institution.

References

1. Chen S, Guan X, Shu Z, Li Y, Cao W, Dong F, Zhang M, Shao G, Shao F. A new application of multimodality radiomics improves diagnostic accuracy of nonpalpable breast lesions in patients with microcalcifications-only in mammography. Med Sci Monit. 2019;20(25):9786–93.
2. Tabár L, Fagerberg CJ, Gad A, Baldetorp L, Holmberg LH, Gröntoft O, Ljungquist U, Lundström B, Månson JC, Eklund G, et al. Reduction in mortality from breast cancer after mass screening with mammography. Randomized trial from the Breast Cancer Screening Working Group of the Swedish National Board of Health and Welfare. Lancet. 1985;1(8433):829–32.
3. Lee CH. Screening mammography: proven benefit, continued controversy. Radiol Clin North Am. 2002;40(3):395–407.
4. Shao J, Rodrigues M, Corter AL, Baxter NN. Multidisciplinary care of breast cancer patients: a scoping review of multidisciplinary styles, processes, and outcomes. Curr Oncol. 2019;26(3):e385–97.

5. Destouet J, Bassett L, Yaffe M, Butler P, Wilcox P. The ACR's mammography accreditation program: ten years of experience since MQSA. JACR. 2005;2(7):585–94.
6. Bassett L, Bent C, Sayre J, Marzan R, Verma A, Porter C. Breast imaging training and attitudes: update survey of senior radiology residents. AJR Am J Roentgenol. 2011;197(1):263–9.
7. Farria D, Salcman J, Monticciolo D, Monses B, Rebner M, Bassett L. A survey of breast imaging fellowship programs: current status of curriculum and training in the United States and Canada. J Am Coll Radiol. 2014;11(9):894–8.
8. Wu T, Law W, Islam N, Yong-Hing CJ, Kulkarni S, Seely J. Factors influencing trainees' interest in breast imaging. Can Assoc Radiol J. 2022;73(3):462–72.
9. Haken OJ, Gong AJ, Ambinder EB, Myers KS, Oluyemi ET. Diversity and inclusion in breast imaging and radiology at large: what can we do to improve? Curr Radiol Rep. 2021;9(12):13.
10. Baxi SS, Liberman L, Lee C, Elkin EB. Breast imaging fellowships in the United States: who, what, and where? AJR Am J Roentgenol. 2009;192(2):403–7.
11. Katzen J, Grimm L, Brem R. The American college of radiology/society of breast imaging updated fellowship training curriculum for breast imaging. J Breast Imaging. 2021;3(4):498–501.
12. https://www.sbi-online.org/breast-imaging-fellowship-match-program#:~:text=The%20 Breast%20Imaging%20Fellowship%20Match,Fellowship%20Match%20for%202024%20 appointments.
13. The Process for Developing ACR Practice Parameters and Technical Standards on the ACR website. https://www.acr.org/Clinical-Resources/Practice-Parameters-and-Technical-Standards by the Committee Practice Parameters – Breast Imaging of the ACR Commission on Breast Imaging. https://www.acr.org/-/media/ACR/Files/Practice-Parameters/screen-diag-mammo.pdf?la=en
14. Monticciolo DL, Rebner M, Appleton CM, et al. The ACR/society of breast imaging resident and fellowship training curriculum for breast imaging, updated. J Am Coll Radiol. 2013;109(3):207–10.
15. Mehta R, Lourenco A, Phillips J. A roadmap for a successful breast imaging fellowship. J Breast Imaging. 2020;2(2):157–60.
16. https://www.nrmp.org/fellowship-applicants/
17. National Resident Matching Program, Results and Data: Specialties Matching Service 2018 Appointment Year. National Resident Matching Program, Washington, DC; 2018.
18. National Resident Matching Program, Results and Data: Specialties Matching Service 2022 Appointment Year. National Resident Matching Program, Washington, DC; 2022.
19. Mullen LA, Nguyen DL, Katzen JT, Brem RF, Ambinder EB. Virtual interviews for breast imaging fellowship during the COVID-19 pandemic: perspectives of program directors and applicants. J Breast Imaging. 2022;4:wbac017.

Chapter 11
Cardiothoracic Imaging Fellowship

Baskaran Sundaram

Introduction

Thoracic radiology in many institutions has evolved into cardiothoracic imaging with the integration of cardiac imaging over the last 20 years. Much of the excitement is due to modern multidetector CT, lung high-resolution CT, dual-energy CT, structural and functional lung and cardiovascular imaging with CT and MRI, and advancement in imaging-guided procedures such as thermal ablation. Chest radiographs are the most common imaging procedure in radiology departments, touching nearly every patient and resulting in up to many hundred thousand patient interactions per year. Similarly, chest CT for thoracic malignancies and angiography for pulmonary embolism and aortic diseases are some of the most commonly performed cross-sectional imaging procedures. Thoracic radiologists are uniquely positioned to handle lung and cardiac diseases, which are almost always intertwined. As a result, cardiothoracic imagers issue high-quality reports in managing expected, unexpected, and incidental cardiothoracic imaging findings. The highly qualitative nature of thoracic imaging is also shifting to more quantitative with population health implications such as COPD, coronary artery calcifications, body composition, and bone mineral density measurements. Thoracic radiology is integral in many large research trials of thoracic diseases, translating into real-life patient care improvements such as early lung cancer detection and coronary atherosclerosis. Recognizing these, many academic departments and radiology organizations have continued to nurture cardiothoracic imaging over the last two to three decades. Increasingly, private practice groups also specifically hire fellowship-trained cardiothoracic radiologists to provide subspecialty-based clinical care to serve their

B. Sundaram (✉)
Thomas Jefferson University Hospital, Philadelphia, PA, USA
e-mail: Baskaran.sundaram@jefferson.edu

J. Shames et al. (eds.), *A Radiologist's Path*,
https://doi.org/10.1007/978-3-031-86882-5_11

59

customers better. Approximately one-third of cardiothoracic imaging fellows directly enter private practice at the end of their fellowship [1].

One of the concerns about cardiac imaging is the turf battle over it. However, the most common arrangement to offer cardiac imaging is a shared service model where cardiology and radiology collaboratively enjoy all aspects of cardiothoracic imaging.

Cardiothoracic Imaging Fellowship Program

Radiology residents enter cardiothoracic imaging fellowship after completing 4 years of radiology residency in the USA. Trainees from outside the USA also enter North American cardiothoracic imaging fellowships. The rules and guidelines for accepting foreign medical graduates vary between institutions and state medical boards. As a result, trainees may receive differing immigration visas from the federal government and restricted or unrestricted medical licensure from the state medical boards. These details are covered in other segments of this book.

Based on a personal survey of the fellowship programs listed on the Society of Thoracic Radiology (STR) website in 2019, more than 53 North American cardiothoracic imaging fellowship programs offer 70 cardiothoracic fellowship positions, each offering one to five fellowship positions per year. Almost all of these programs are in academic medical centers. Programs may call the fellowships cardiothoracic or cardiac and pulmonary or chest or thoracic imaging fellowships. Although all are expected to have a structure, all of the cardiothoracic imaging fellowships in the USA currently do not have CAQ accreditation.

Structure

The structure of a cardiothoracic imaging fellowship varies between institutions. The most common structure is appropriately portioned thoracic and cardiac imaging modalities (rarely, including nuclear medicine) and image-guided procedures for 12 consecutive months. Some programs may allow dedicated nonclinical days for research and educational activities. Programs may offer exposure in abdominal, nuclear medicine, musculoskeletal, breast imaging, informatics, echocardiography, and radiology technologist rotation. Since these components' ratio, frequency, duration, and contiguity may vary, many creatively organize their fellowship experience.

Fellows may provide patient care outside regular business hours, solely in cardiothoracic imaging or combined with other imaging specialties. Faculty will directly supervise the cardiothoracic imaging fellows. Fellows may only function as trainees during their fellowship or enjoy optimal autonomy. The departments may titrate the fellows' supervision level during the fellowship year. Hence, institutions may provide fellows with medical school appointments as a lecturer.

Cardiothoracic imaging fellows will be encouraged to participate in multidisciplinary clinical conferences such as thoracic oncology, interstitial lung disease, and cardiovascular conferences. There will be opportunities to teach the students and residents in the reading room and didactic conferences. Fellows may champion conferences on interesting or challenging diagnoses and quality improvement. Although clinical care and education are the mainstays of the cardiothoracic imaging fellowship, departments encourage and support fellows performing research, presenting at national conferences, and publishing.

Curriculum

Cardiothoracic fellowship programs mirror STR's core curriculum covering a variety of thoracic diseases using all available imaging modalities, most commonly using chest radiographs, CT, MRI, and rarely PET scans [2]. Fellows receive informal teaching at the workstation and formal periodic educational lectures in thoracic imaging in combination with department-wide teaching activities for all radiology fellows. Fellowship programs may partner with an external program to address specific educational needs. Fellowship programs may adopt a supercharged curriculum version if they mutually decide on an abbreviated fellowship. Also, during the last year of radiology residency, programs offer customizable and focused mini fellowships in cardiothoracic imaging training that may last weeks to months to prepare residents for the next chapter in functioning as independent radiologists. Cardiothoracic fellowship programs will have periodic meetings with the fellowship director to evaluate the strengths and weaknesses of the program and trainees and document competence. At the end of the fellowship, fellows may receive certifications and are encouraged to have documentation of their work volumes, teaching case collection, and procedure logs to support their future workplace privileges applications, such as level 2 and 3 advanced cardiac imaging.

An improved understanding of cardiac pathophysiology is essential to obtain diagnostic quality cardiothoracic imaging examination. The cardiac techs are often knowledgeable in tweaking the scan parameters and improving the examination's diagnostic yield. Hence, fellows are encouraged to learn by being physically present in the scanning suite and functioning as technologists to perform cardiac CT/MRI examinations. Also, image post-processing is an essential aspect of cardiothoracic imaging. Hence, learning from the super technologists or 3D image post-processing labs is also encouraged. Institutions may offer hands-on learning experiences through simulation labs to become proficient in image-guided procedures.

Due to the close involvement in managing contrast reactions, interventional procedures, and administering cardiac medications for CT, departments encourage and sponsor fellows to obtain BLS and ACLS certifications.

Clinical Workflow and Artificial Intelligence

The cardiothoracic imaging division may share its services with other groups, for example, chest X-ray with MSK and community radiology, cardiac imaging with cardiologists, chest CT with emergency or body or community radiology, and thoracic imaging-guided interventions with interventional radiology. Various reasons dictate the differences in these ever-growing workloads and demands. Hence, understanding the local workflow will benefit the cardiothoracic imaging fellows. There may also be moonlighting opportunities outside the regular work hours.

Cardiothoracic imaging fellows will interface with artificial intelligence/machine learning (AI/ML) tools during the fellowship. As of October 2022, 75% of 521 FDA-approved AI/ML tools are focused on radiology, and cardiology comes at a distant second place at 10% [3]. These tools are more prevalent in cardiothoracic imaging than in other parts of radiology. They range from detecting lung nodules and pneumothorax to accelerating image acquisition, analysis, and reporting.

Society of Thoracic Radiology (STR)

STR is a thriving organization and an excellent professional home since 1982 to many thoracic radiologists worldwide. It offers free memberships for trainees. The STR actively maintains its website with content on education, annual meetings, mentoring, newsletter, membership details, research, the society's official journal, fellowships, social media links, intersociety relationships, and career opportunities [4]. The STR website links various fellowship programs, contact information, and a sample application form. The STR's annual meeting is during the spring months, and the venue changes yearly. Both virtual and in-person attendances are possible. During this meeting, speakers worldwide lecture on various cardiothoracic imaging topics. Cardiothoracic imaging fellows find the annual meetings inspirational to witness experts lecturing and interacting with them. Fellows also enjoy presenting at this meeting ranging from case-of-the-day presentations to poster and oral abstract presentations and lectures. Fellows are encouraged to attend informal gatherings during this meeting and enjoy networking opportunities. Fellows are also eligible for travel grants.

The cardiothoracic imaging community is close-knit. As a result, it is easier for cardiothoracic imaging fellows to receive many aspects of mentoring. Currently, the STR offers to mentor junior faculty launching their career as cardiothoracic radiologists addressing various topics such as enhancing clinical skills, teaching, networking, scholarly activities, and work-life balance.

Conclusion

Cardiothoracic imaging is an excellent radiology specialty interacting with clinicians managing intertwined cardiac and lung diseases. Cardiothoracic radiologists issue valuable imaging reports. Cardiothoracic imaging fellowships offer an opportunity to customize and maximize the learning potential. AI tools are increasingly prevalent and promising in cardiothoracic imaging and may become mainstream to facilitate quantitative imaging. To top it off, the close-knit, collaborative cardiothoracic imaging community offers excellent networking and a long and gratifying career.

References

1. Society of Thoracic Radiology Website. https://thoracicrad.org/?page_id=162
2. Gilman MD, et al. Hybrid PET/CT of the thorax: when is computer registration necessary? J Comput Assist Tomogr. 2007;31(3):395–401.
3. Retrieved from https://www.fda.gov/medical-devices/software-medical-device-samd/artificial-intelligence-and-machine-learning-aiml-enabled-medical-devices?
4. Retrieved from https://thoracicrad.org/

Chapter 12
Fellowship in Cardiovascular Imaging

Tessa S. Cook

Introduction

If you enjoy imaging of the heart and vascular anatomy, advanced image processing, optimizing protocols according to vascular anatomy and physiology, and multiple opportunities to innovate, you should consider a fellowship in cardiovascular imaging (CVI). Advanced training in cardiac imaging for radiologists is often bundled with either thoracic (cardiothoracic) or vascular (cardiovascular) imaging. The Society for Thoracic Radiology maintains a list of cardiothoracic radiology training programs [1], and the North American Society for Cardiovascular Imaging maintains a list of cardiovascular imaging fellowships [2]. At present in the United States, there are many more cardiothoracic fellowships than cardiovascular fellowships.

Benefits of a Cardiovascular Imaging Fellowship

Radiology residents typically do not have much exposure to cardiac imaging during their training. At many centers, the cardiac imaging service is run exclusively by cardiology or as a collaboration between radiology and cardiology. As such, most radiology residents must pursue fellowship training to get in-depth experience in cardiac imaging. Vascular imaging—with computed tomography (CT) angiography and magnetic resonance (MR) angiography, generally remains within radiology departments. In departments without a dedicated cardiovascular division,

T. S. Cook (✉)
Department of Radiology, Perelman School of Medicine at the University of Pennsylvania, Philadelphia, PA, USA
e-mail: tessa.cook@pennmedicine.upenn.edu

© The Author(s), under exclusive license to Springer Nature Switzerland AG 2025
J. Shames et al. (eds.), *A Radiologist's Path*,
https://doi.org/10.1007/978-3-031-86882-5_12

abdominal radiologists or vascular/interventional radiologists typically interpret these cases. Emergency radiology divisions also cover these types of cases.

Dedicated training in cardiovascular or cardiothoracic imaging provides advanced training in processing and interpreting complex imaging of the heart and vasculature. Fellowship-trained cardiovascular radiologists are often responsible for interpreting multiple imaging modalities to guide patient management and procedural planning. In many instances, patients will undergo imaging with CT, MR, and nuclear cardiology, making this multimodality knowledge critical to deliver high-quality patient care.

Unique Aspects of Cardiovascular Imaging Fellowship Training

In addition to learning how to interpret these cases, cardiovascular imaging fellows also learn how to perform sometimes-complex exams and optimize them to each patient, whether adult or pediatric. Unlike in other areas of diagnostic radiology, cardiovascular radiologists may monitor certain exams while in progress and make necessary adjustments to the protocols. Patients' heart rates, rhythms, and comorbidities, such as congenital heart disease, heart failure, arrhythmias, or the presence of a pacemaker or defibrillator, can affect protocol planning. Protocol optimization for cardiovascular imaging necessitates both a keen understanding of imaging physics and the unique anatomy and physiology of the patient. In cardiovascular CT, the amount and timing of intravenous contrast must be carefully considered. In cardiovascular MR, real-time interpretation of sequences already obtained may inform the addition of other pulse sequences to better answer the clinical question.

Components of Fellowship Training

Cardiovascular imaging fellowship training involves learning about anatomy, physiology, pathophysiology, imaging modalities, and treatments relevant to the field.

The most common cardiac imaging modalities include:

- Cardiac and vascular CT angiography (CTA).
- Cardiac MR imaging (MRI) without and with stress.
- Vascular MR angiography (MRA).
- Nuclear cardiology—including cardiac positron emission tomography (PET), single-photon emission computerized tomography (SPECT), and planar imaging without and with stress.
- Echocardiography.[1]

---

[1] Typically performed and interpreted by cardiologists rather than radiologists

- Cardiac catheterization.[2]

Learning and applying the relevant imaging principles of the modalities above is a crucial part of cardiovascular fellowship training. Knowing how to identify and address artifacts in imaging, recognizing the limitations of each modality in certain situations, and understanding how to tailor an imaging examination to answer a clinical question are important aspects of advanced training in cardiovascular imaging.

In addition to the acquisition modalities listed above, there is substantial post-processing of acquired images for both qualitative and quantitative purposes. At large quaternary medical centers, this may be performed by a standalone 3D lab [3]; nevertheless, cardiovascular radiologists must also be proficient in analyzing and processing these cases. Fellowship training includes gaining this proficiency with a variety of case types and software applications. Examples of post-processing are shown in Figs. 12.1 and 12.2.

A major component of training is becoming familiar with the various cardiovascular diseases and therapeutic procedures for which imaging is indicated. This includes complex cardiovascular anatomy and variants that can occur before/after birth, as well as their associated appearances after medical management/surgical correction. Table 12.1 describes some of the important conditions and procedures that should be learned during fellowship.

Other aspects of fellowship training include:

- Exposure to cardiac imaging outside of radiology, such as echocardiography, cardiac catheterization, and nuclear cardiology.

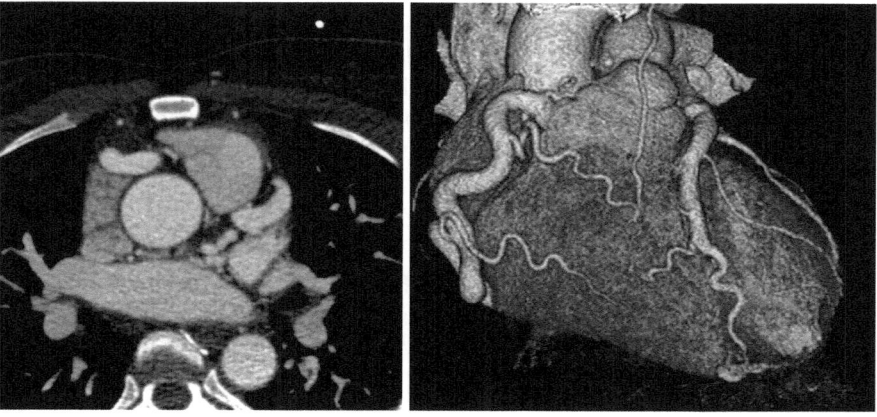

Fig. 12.1 Patient with unrepaired anomalous left coronary artery arising from the pulmonary artery (ALCAPA). (Left) axial CTA image showing dilated, tortuous coronary arteries. (Right) 3D volume rendering from the same CTA also showing collaterals between the left and right coronary arteries

---

[2] Almost exclusively performed and interpreted by cardiologists

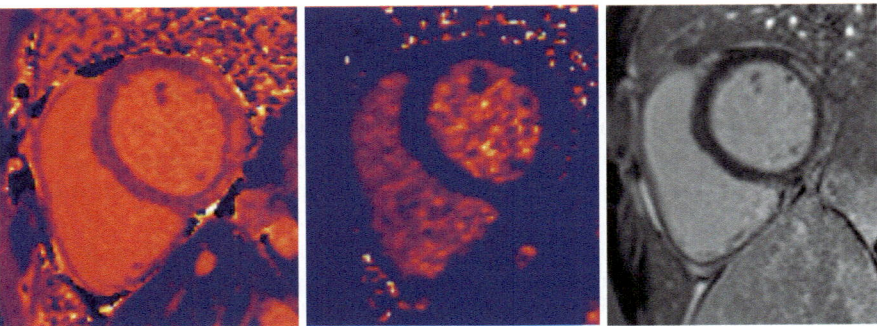

Fig. 12.2 Tissue characterization with cardiac MRI in a patient with COVID-19 myocarditis. (Left) native T1 map showing high myocardial T1 in the mid-myocardial to subepicardial lateral wall of the left ventricle. (Middle) T2 map showing myocardial edema in the same segments. (Right) late gadolinium enhancement (LGE) image showing increased signal in the same segments

Table 12.1 Categories and examples of disease processes and therapeutic options with which cardiovascular radiologists should be familiar

Aortic disease	Heart disease	Coronary artery disease	Procedural planning
Acute aortic injury	Ischemic heart disease	Stenosis	Ablation
Aortic surgical planning	Nonischemic cardiomyopathies	Plaque characterization	Transcatheter valve replacement
Postoperative aorta and complications	Genetic cardiomyopathies	Anatomic variants	Open vs. endovascular aortic repair
Congenital variants	Congenital heart disease	Postoperative appearance	Flap planning
Vasculitides	Structural heart disease		

- Exposure to cardiac inpatient and outpatient services to understand the symptoms, clinical presentation, and initial workup that leads to cardiovascular imaging.
- Exposure to vascular surgery.
- Participation in multidisciplinary conferences.

Each of these experiences provides further advanced training in the field that both informs and complements interpretation of cardiovascular imaging.

Advanced Certifications in Cardiovascular Imaging

There are multiple advanced certifications in cardiovascular imaging attainable during or soon after fellowship. These credentials support the expertise of the fellows and new practitioners of cardiovascular imaging and attest to the level of experience they have in the field.

Guidelines from the SCCT published in 2020 describe the education and experience qualifications necessary to achieve independent practitioner (formerly Level II) or advanced practitioner (formerly Level III) certification in cardiovascular CT [4]. Independent practitioners have achieved competency to independently protocol and interpret cardiac CT as well as evaluate common anatomy and pathology on cardiac CT, including basic congenital heart disease. In addition to these competencies, advanced practitioners can also evaluate complex cardiac and congenital heart disease and vascular disease on CT and are qualified to lead a clinical cardiovascular laboratory with appropriate accreditation, equipment, quality improvement, and administrative knowledge.

Analogous guidelines from the SCMR published in 2018 are also available for training in cardiovascular MR [5]. Level 2 training qualifies a physician to independently perform and interpret cardiovascular MR, while Level 3 training is suitable for physicians who wish to run a cardiovascular MR laboratory.

Certification is available for both cardiovascular CT and MR through the Certification Board of Cardiovascular CT (CBCCT™) and the Certification Board of Cardiovascular MR (CBCMR™). Information about these certifications is available online.

Professional Societies

Several professional societies are dedicated to cardiovascular imaging. These include the following:

- Society for Cardiovascular Computed Tomography (SCCT).
  - http://www.scct.org
- Society for Cardiovascular Magnetic Resonance (SCMR).
  - http://www.scmr.org
- North American Society for Cardiovascular Imaging (NASCI).
  - http://www.nasci.org
- Society for Thoracic Radiology (STR).
  - http://www.str.org
- American Heart Association (AHA).
  - http://www.aha.org

References

1. Society for Thoracic Radiology. Cardiothoracic Imaging Fellowship Directory. https://thoracicrad.org/?page_id=318. Accessed 8 June 2023.
2. North American Society for Cardiovascular Imaging. Fellowship Programs. https://nasci.org/resources/fellowship/. Accessed 8 June 2023.
3. Cook TS, Stengall SJ, Steingall SR, Boonn WW. Establishing and running a three-dimensional and advanced imaging laboratory. Radiographics. 2018;38(6):1799–809.
4. Choi AD, Thomas DM, Lee J, et al. 2020 SCCT guideline for training cardiology and radiology trainees as independent practitioners (level II) and advanced practitioners (level III) in cardiovascular computed tomography: a statement from the Society of Cardiovascular Computed Tomography. J Cardiovasc Comput Tomogr. 2021;15(1):2–15. https://doi.org/10.1016/j.jcct.2020.08.003.
5. Kim RJ, Simonetti OP, Westwood M, et al. Guidelines for training in cardiovascular magnetic resonance (CMR). J Cardiovasc Magn Reson. 2018;20:57. https://doi.org/10.1186/s12968-018-0481-8.

Chapter 13
Emergency Radiology

Amy Haberman

Because of the various modalities and pathologies in the emergency room, radiologists must be ready to interpret them all. Those that staff these divisions have become the new "general" radiologist. Depending on the hospital size and number of patients serviced through emergency rooms, some emergency radiologists are subspecialized within the emergency division. Some may read everything, and some may be divided into body radiologists, neuroradiologists, or variations.

Because of this growing specialty, the American Society of Emergency Radiology was created in 1988. In 1995, the society started the journal *Emergency Radiology*, a peer-reviewed journal of practical imaging. The society also helps to advance the specialty and improve radiologic aspects of emergency care, helps develop educational curricula for medical students and residents, acts as a resource for those who practice emergency radiology, and creates a standard of care within the field.

Currently, there are 21 emergency radiology fellowships in the United States. These consist of 12 months of training, each program uniquely designed to provide the fellow opportunities to learn according to their interests.

The greatest draws to this subspecialty are the variety of cases and scheduled shift work. Most emergency radiologists have set hours and usually do not take call, similar to emergency room physicians. The drawback is that emergency radiology is a 24-h service; therefore, night shifts are typically required.

Emergency radiologists face challenges that include understanding all emergency processes from head to toe and recognizing these pathologies promptly with many interruptions and unpredictable case volumes.

A. Haberman (✉)
Department of Radiology, NYU Grossman School of Medicine, New Hyde Park, NY, USA

J. Shames et al. (eds.), *A Radiologist's Path*,
https://doi.org/10.1007/978-3-031-86882-5_13

In conclusion, this rapidly growing subspecialty provides interpretive expertise with the most incredible variety of cases, appealing to many radiology trainees. It offers around-the-clock coverage in hospital settings and has come to work hand in hand with emergency room physicians to provide fast, high-quality care that all patients need.

Chapter 14
Fellowship in Imaging Informatics

Tessa S. Cook

Introduction

Do you identify a problem in the reading room or your clinical workflow and wish you could solve it? You might have the makings of an imaging informaticist! Imaging informatics is the specialty that considers the human-computer interfaces in medical imaging and the workflow, standards, challenges, and opportunities to improve healthcare using technology. Fellowship training in imaging informatics is now available to both radiology residents finishing their training and radiologists in practice looking to advance their skills and proficiency. A variety of program structures exist to accommodate fellows at different career levels.

Although imaging informatics spans a variety of clinical disciplines, including radiology, cardiology, pathology, dermatology, ophthalmology, dentistry, and more, we will focus our discussion on its role in diagnostic radiology.

Imaging Informatics Versus Clinical Informatics

The fields of imaging informatics and clinical informatics are very closely related [1]. Both deal with the domain of patient care and systems that interact with one another [2]. However, imaging informatics focuses on the clinical systems that deal specifically with image acquisition, display, postprocessing, and imaging reporting, such as the following:

T. S. Cook (✉)
Department of Radiology, Perelman School of Medicine at the University of Pennsylvania, Philadelphia, PA, USA
e-mail: tessa.cook@pennmedicine.upenn.edu

© The Author(s), under exclusive license to Springer Nature
Switzerland AG 2025
J. Shames et al. (eds.), *A Radiologist's Path*,
https://doi.org/10.1007/978-3-031-86882-5_14

- Picture archiving and communications system (PACS).
- Radiology information system (RIS).
- Dictation/voice recognition software.

Nevertheless, these systems interact closely with the electronic medical record, which is the workhorse of clinical informatics, and the patient portal.

Radiologists use other software applications in different areas of practice, and these must also be integrated into the clinical workflow in as seamless a fashion as possible. Imaging informaticists are responsible for these integrations as well as others and manage the flow of patient data between systems used for care delivery.

Benefits of an Imaging Informatics Fellowship

In years past, imaging informatics was primarily taught in residency programs that had a high concentration of experts in the field. In 2016, radiology leaders realized the value of imaging informatics and the importance of teaching the fundamentals of this field to all radiology residents, not just those with access to experts. As a result of this discussion, the National Imaging Informatics Course (NIIC) was developed as a collaboration between the RSNA and SIIM (Society for Imaging Informatics in Medicine), with the support of the Association of Academic Radiology (AAR) [3]. The NIIC continues to serve as an introductory course in the field, allowing participants to build on the fundamental concepts taught during a subsequent imaging informatics fellowship. There are more than a dozen imaging informatics fellowship programs across the United States, all of which have a unique structure [4].

An informatics fellowship gives you the ability to gain advanced training in a field that is in high demand, [5], particularly in recent years as investment in artificial intelligence (AI) in medical imaging has burgeoned. As radiologists, we interact with several hardware and software systems throughout our clinical day. The complex interactions between radiologists and computer systems, as well as between different computer systems, may seem mysterious sometimes, especially when something does not work as expected. Informaticists understand these interactions and can more effectively design systems that work together, troubleshoot problems, and develop innovative solutions.

Informatics fellows get to look under the hood of common systems used in radiology, such as PACS, RIS, dictation/reporting software, other radiology postprocessing applications, AI models, large language models (LLMs), and their connections to the electronic medical record (EMR). As an informatics fellow, you will learn about the international standards that govern interoperability of clinical systems, such as the following:

- DICOM: Digital Imaging and Communications in Medicine.

    (a) For exchange, display, storage, and output of medical images.

- HL7: Health Level 7.

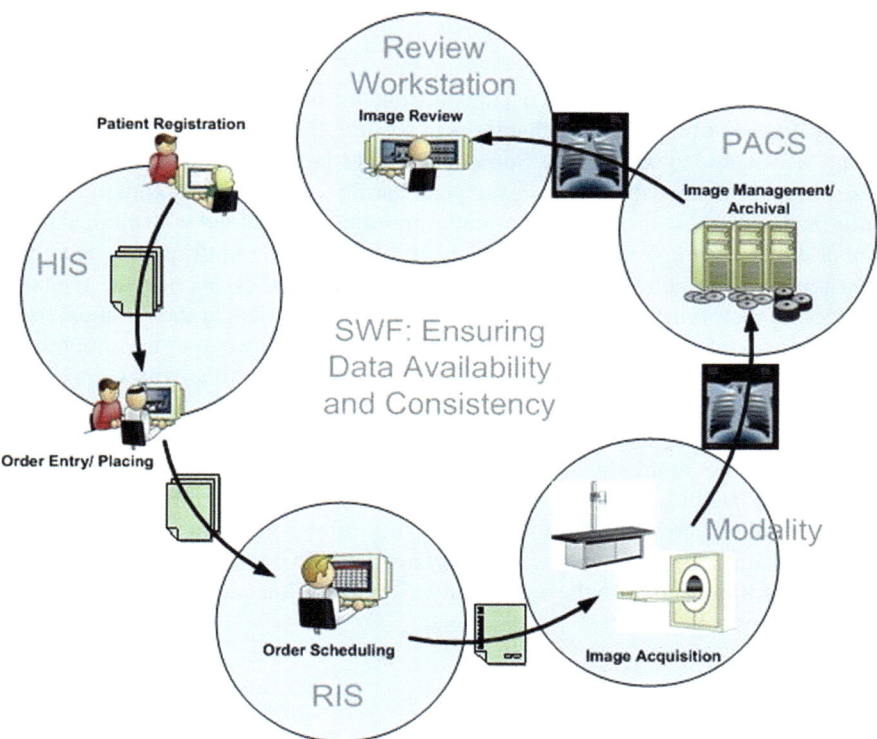

Fig. 14.1 Scheduled Workflow (SWF) integration profile from IHE®. Available at https://wiki. ihe.net/index.php/Scheduled_Workflow

(b) For exchange of *other* medical data, such as in the EMR.

- HL7 FHIR: HL7 Fast Healthcare Interoperability Resources.

(c) For exchange of medical data using internet-based transactions.

Figure 14.1 demonstrates an early example of radiology workflow and systems interoperability. It illustrates the Scheduled Workflow (SWF) profile developed by the Integrating the Healthcare Enterprise (IHE®) initiative, an international collaboration dedicated to improving interoperability of clinical systems across healthcare (not just in medical imaging).

As AI applications continue to permeate medicine, there are even more systems that could enter the clinical radiology workflow and even more need for imaging informaticists to be involved in designing, selecting, implementing, and monitoring this new technology [6].

Fellowship Structure Options

Of the approximately one dozen clinical imaging informatics fellowships in the United States at the time this chapter was written, there are a variety of program formats available to fellows [4]. Some fellowships are fully dedicated to informatics, where the fellow spends the entire year learning about and working in imaging informatics. In most instances, informatics training is combined with clinical training or clinical work. Fellows may spend half of their time in informatics and cover that time with evening or overnight call. Alternatively, they may spend a smaller fraction of their time on informatics training as a complement to their clinical training. For example, fellows may meet for a few hours each week or each month for focused informatics training and supplement that in-person time with independent study and individual projects in between in-person sessions.

In addition to clinical fellowships, there are also informatics master's programs that follow more traditional academic schedules. These programs may fall under the umbrella of health informatics or bioinformatics and typically offer a comprehensive curriculum across multiple semesters. They often address far more than imaging informatics. These programs generally require a final thesis or capstone project that provides students with the opportunity to apply the knowledge they have gained from the program.

Components of Fellowship Training

Informatics fellowships involve multiple types of educational experiences (Table 14.1). They typically include didactic sessions from experts on a particular topic. In this heavily connected world, the experts are not necessarily faculty at the same institution at which the fellowship is conducted. Most fellowships include discussion sessions, either structured around a journal article or a particular set of themes. Many fellowships also include hands-on lab sessions, where fellows gain experience with programming, AI, or informatics tools such as an open-source PACS, HL7/FHIR application programmer interfaces (APIs), network monitoring/ optimization tools, etc. Joint sessions between fellowship programs and a national

Table 14.1 Topics often covered in imaging informatics fellowships [7]

Imaging informatics fellowship topics		
Computers and networking	Artificial intelligence	Business of imaging informatics
Standards and interoperability	Enterprise imaging	Artificial intelligence
Workflow	Privacy and security	Natural language processing
PACS/RIS	Business intelligence	Informatics outside of radiology
Governance	Data science	Education
Regulation and legislation	Ethics	Quality and safety

session sponsored by SIIM for all informatics fellowships are also available as supplemental educational experiences.

Imaging Informatics Specialty Societies

Several professional societies are dedicated to imaging informatics and/or clinical informatics. These include the following:

- Society for Imaging Informatics in Medicine (SIIM).

    - http://www.siim.org
- Health Information Management and Systems Society (HIMSS).

    - http://www.himss.org
- European Society for Medical Imaging Informatics (EuSoMII).

    - http://www.eusomii.org
    - Closely aligned with SIIM.
- Radiological Society of North America (RSNA).

    - http://www.rsna.org/
- American College of Radiology (ACR).

    - https://www.acr.org/Data-Science-and-Informatics/Informatics
    - ACR Data Science Institute: https://www.acr.org/data-science-and-informatics/ACR-Data-Science-Institute
- American Medical Informatics Association (AMIA).

    - http://www.amia.org

Specialty Certifications in Imaging Informatics

The American Board of Imaging Informatics (ABII) offers the Certified Imaging Informatics Professional (CIIP) licensure to qualified candidates. Radiologists are qualified to apply at the end of the first year of radiology residency. As with other board certifications, there is a 10-year recertification process with multiple pathways. Information is available online at http://www.abii.org.

The American Board of Preventative Medicine (ABPM) offers a clinical informatics board certification to eligible physicians who have demonstrated a commitment to clinical informatics work. Clinical informatics board certification includes some imaging informatics but is heavily focused on other concepts, including clinical decision support, EMR optimization, leadership and project management, and enterprise information systems. At the time of this chapter writing, there are two pathways for eligibility: the Practice Pathway and the Accreditation Council for Graduate Medical Education (ACGME)-Accredited Fellowship Pathway. Beginning in 2026, only the Fellowship Pathway will be offered. Specific details are available at https://www.theabpm.org/become-certified/subspecialties/clinical-informatics/.

References

1. Whitfill JT, Kalpas E, Garcia-Filion P. Reuniting long lost cousins: a novel curriculum in imaging informatics for clinical informatics fellows. J Digit Imaging. 2022;35(4):876–80. https://doi.org/10.1007/s10278-022-00628-5.
2. Bumbarger NA, Towbin AJ, Garcia-Filion P, et al. Imaging Informatics Education in Clinical Informatics Programs: Perspective from Imaging and Clinical Informatics Professionals. Appl Clin Inform. 2024 Aug;15(4):756–62. https://doi.org/10.1055/s-0044-1788327.
3. National Imaging Informatics Course – The NIIC. https://siim.org/learning-events/learning/niic/. Accessed 29 Aug 2023.
4. Imaging Informatics Fellowship Programs. https://siim.org/resources/imaging-informatics-fellowship/. Accessed 29 Aug 2023.
5. Vey BL, Cook TS, Nagy P, et al. A survey of imaging informatics fellowships and their curricula: current state assessment. J Digit Imaging. 2019;32(1):91–6. https://doi.org/10.1007/s10278-018-0147-y.
6. Cook TS. The importance of imaging informatics and Informaticists in the implementation of AI. Acad Rad. 2020;27(1):113–6. https://doi.org/10.1016/j.acra.2019.10.002.
7. Gerard R, Makeeva V, Vey B, et al. Imaging informatics fellowship curriculum: building consensus on the most critical topics and the future of the informatics fellowship. J Digit Imaging. 2023;36(1):1–10. https://doi.org/10.1007/s10278-022-00702-y.

Chapter 15
Musculoskeletal (MSK) Fellowship

Evan Rochlis and Jeffrey A. Belair

Application Process

Musculoskeletal (MSK) radiology is a one-year fellowship for graduates of radiology residency. Applicants typically apply during PGY4/R3 year via the musculoskeletal radiology fellowship match, which is governed by the Society of Skeletal Radiology (SSR) (https://skeletalrad.org/) and administered by the National Resident Matching Program (NRMP) (https://www.nrmp.org/). As of the 2024 match year, 78 MSK fellowship programs participated in the match according to the NRMP [1]. These programs are a mix between ACGME-accredited fellowships and nonaccredited fellowships, with the details of each program listed on their respective websites. The differences between ACGME and non-ACGME fellowships are negligible to most applicants, with the most significant implications for those on visa sponsorship. Programs offer between one and nine fellowship positions per year.

The SSR publishes a timeline for the match each year. Most programs accept a common application form provided by the SSR. However, some programs may instead require an internal application, usually found on their fellowship websites. The MSK match, which abides by the Society of Chairs of Academic Radiology Departments (SCARD) embargo, currently allows programs to begin accepting applications on November 1. Interviews can start in early-mid January and must be completed by the end of March [2]. The NRMP then allows trainees and programs to construct rank lists in mid April. Final rank list submissions are due at the beginning of June, and the match is typically two weeks later.

To be a competitive applicant, thoroughly preparing for the match process is best. Securing three strong letters of recommendation, including at least one from a musculoskeletal radiologist, is an early priority. Hence, faculty have enough time to

E. Rochlis · J. A. Belair (✉)
Thomas Jefferson University, Philadelphia, PA, USA
e-mail: evan.rochlis@jefferson.edu; jeffrey.belair@jefferson.edu

© The Author(s), under exclusive license to Springer Nature
Switzerland AG 2025
J. Shames et al. (eds.), *A Radiologist's Path*,
https://doi.org/10.1007/978-3-031-86882-5_15

79

write a letter before the application cycle commences. Once applications open, submitting applications early on will demonstrate that the candidate is prepared and decisive. Future candidates should consider following the SSR as soon as they are interested in the MSK radiology fellowship. In addition to providing educational content in MSK radiology on their website, the SSR regularly hosts webinars targeted to trainees, including an "MSK Fellowship Panel." The annual SSR meeting is held in March at various locations across the United States. While this meeting had previously been closed to residents, it now includes a special resident session open to SSR scholars and those residents whose work has been accepted for presentation. The annual SSR meeting provides an opportunity to network within the relatively tight-knit subspeciality and attend lectures by leading MSK faculty nationwide.

The data from the NRMP for the 2024 Match demonstrates a match rate of 98.7% with a total of 58 unfilled fellowship positions across 35 MSK radiology programs (see table below) [1]. Thus, most applicants can count on finding a spot within the match if they apply widely and are reasonably qualified. Applicants will benefit from strong letters of recommendation, well-written personal statements, and polished interview skills regarding matching at their top program.

Applicant statistics	Number	%
Matched applicants	156	
US foreign	9	5.8
MD graduate	99	63.5
Foreign graduate	14	9.0
DO graduate	33	21.2
Total matched	156	98.7
Total unmatched	2	1.3
Program statistics	Number	%
Certified programs	78	
Programs filled	43	55.1
Programs unfilled	35	44.9
Certified positions	214	
Positions filled	156	72.9
Positions unfilled	58	27.1

Fellowship Training

For ACGME-accredited programs, the SSR publishes a comprehensive list of requirements for fellowships to help standardize subspecialty training. Responsibilities for an MSK radiology fellow must include these six items:

1. Protocoling, monitoring, and interpreting CT and MR imaging studies under faculty supervision

2. Protocoling and performing patient procedures, including arthrography, therapeutic and diagnostic injections, ultrasound, and CT-guided biopsies under faculty supervision
3. Performing diagnostic MSK ultrasound examinations and presenting the findings to the attending for review
4. Preparing interdisciplinary conferences
5. Consulting with referring physicians
6. Effectively communicating study results by timely signing of reports and appropriate direct communication

Diagnostic responsibilities include protocoling and interpreting both musculoskeletal CT and MRI. Fellows must learn to perform and interpret diagnostic musculoskeletal ultrasounds. Procedural skills learned during fellowship include procedures performed under CT, ultrasound, and fluoroscopic guidance. Participating in interdisciplinary conferences is a requirement and can be satisfied in many fields: orthopedic oncology, sarcoma tumor board, pathology, sports medicine, rheumatology, or any other combination of disciplines. The *ACGME-required* responsibilities of a fellow in MSK radiology do not include any calls. However, most programs will require some amount of call.

In addition to the responsibilities of the fellows to interpret findings and perform procedures, each fellowship program is tasked with educating fellows by providing a robust didactic curriculum covering the following topics:

- Common fractures of the axial and appendicular skeleton (including mechanisms of injury and potential complications)
- Orthopedic appliances and hardware used to fixate these fractures and their complications
- Bone and soft tissue tumors (using the WHO classification system), both for initial presentation and recurrent and metastatic disease assessment
- Osteonecrosis
- Metabolic bone disease
- Arthropathies (degenerative, inflammatory, and crystal)
- Systemic disorders to include hematopoietic and storage diseases
- Abnormalities of the knee, shoulder, foot, ankle, hand, wrist, hip, and pelvis
- Disorders of the spine (including disc pathology using the ASNR nomenclature)

Throughout the year, fellows are required by the ACGME to undergo regular assessments in various educational and professional domains by their peers and faculty [3]. At the end of the fellowship, the program must submit a summative fellow evaluation for graduation. There are no strict case number requirements that programs are bound to graduate fellows, but instead, they are expected to acquire the requisite knowledge to serve as MSK subspecialty consultants by the end of their training year. There is no in-training or subspecialty board examination for MSK radiologists, but they must become certified by the American Board of Radiology (ABR) after graduation. Fellow responsibilities and the academic requirements for ACGME programs do not apply to non-ACGME-accredited fellowships. While the ACGME offers suggested guidelines for non-ACGME fellowships, these fellowships are not bound to adhere to a strict curriculum.

What to Look for in a Program

The regular duties of an MSK radiologist will differ based on the needs of their practice, and there is wide variability in training strengths and weaknesses among fellowships. To succeed in finding the right fellowship, applicants should consider what skills they would value acquiring most in training that they can bring to their practice after fellowship.

A future career in academia emphasizing publishing can benefit from training in a highly academic program. By looking at the academic output from fellows in years past and from the attendings within a program, one can get a sense of whether the program would prepare them for a job in an academic setting. Applicants may want a program with dedicated research time either weekly or in a block to focus on research before starting their career as an attending.

The number of faculty, number of fellows, and faculty/fellow ratio will impact training. A large group of fellows can divide responsibilities and share learning through case conferences or journal club meetings. However, if cases or procedures are limited, having too many fellows competing for volume may negatively impact the learning process. The number of residents and frequency of resident MRI rotations may also affect the available case volume.

One of the most critical considerations in training is volume. Seeing many subspecialty cases is essential to building accuracy and speed as a fellow enters practice. The ACGME offers no requirements for the number of MSK MRI and CT cases interpreted during the fellowship [4]. An applicant should inquire about the volume of MRI and CT expected to be interpreted daily, the volume of outpatient, inpatient, and emergency cases, and how frequent and detailed readouts are with the attendings. Many trainees have limited exposure to advanced MSK imaging in residency and may want to target programs where fellows have graduated responsibilities for the volume of interpretation throughout the year. Pediatric imaging is not an ACGME requirement for MSK radiology fellowships. However, it may be included as a feature of some programs.

While the ACGME does not require programs to offer training in musculoskeletal radiography, interpretation of radiographs can play a prominent role in some fellowships and be virtually nonexistent in others (except as a reference when interpreting MRI and CT). Whether you wish to have more exposure to radiographs may depend on your residency training and your expectations for a career. Most private practice radiologists will be expected to read radiographs rapidly.

The number and types of procedures a fellow must perform during the year are not specified by the ACGME [4]. All trainees in MSK radiology should be skilled in performing arthrograms and arthrocentesis, as this is a widely used skill that will likely be needed both in private practice and academia. The number and complexity of CT-guided biopsy cases vary between institutions depending on whether the facility is a sizeable tertiary-care referral center for orthopedic oncology. Similarly, ultrasound-guided joint injections are often performed by radiologists, anesthesia/pain physicians, rheumatologists, and sports medicine doctors; therefore, the distribution of cases and volume will vary among institutions. Likewise, spinal epidural and nerve root injections are common pain procedures that pain medicine physicians, sports medicine physicians, and radiologists perform. The ACGME does not require training in these procedures but may be included as a part of fellowship training in some programs. Depending on the institution, IR, neuroradiology, or MSK radiology may perform advanced image-guided procedures such as vertebroplasty, kyphoplasty, and CT-guided tumor ablations. Trainees should target programs based on their comfort with these procedures and their desire to include them in their future practice.

Finally, lifestyle will be an essential factor in any career decision. The physical location usually plays a significant role in fellowship selection. Many trainees have family ties to locations, and moving away for a year can be difficult. If you intend to work in a specific place, choosing a fellowship at a well-known program in the area can be an excellent way to jump-start the job search process. Call can also significantly impact lifestyle during fellowship and will vary across programs. While there are few MSK emergencies, each program will treat call responsibilities differently based on the needs and resources on weekends and holidays.

Lifestyle

Musculoskeletal radiology can be an immensely fulfilling subspecialty. Compared to their radiology peers, MSK radiologists typically enjoy regular work hours, fewer emergent cases, and proportionally greater outpatient studies. Most image-guided MSK procedures performed by MSK radiologists are reasonably quick and gratifying, with the ability to perform more complex vertebral augmentation and tumor ablation procedures if desired. Furthermore, MSK radiologists often have a close working relationship with orthopedic surgeons and sports medicine physicians, which can provide opportunities for interdisciplinary collaboration. Like other radiology subspecialties, MSK radiologists' earnings are on par with the average compensation reported in the 2024 Medscape Radiologist Compensation Report as $498,000 [5].

A musculoskeletal radiologist's day-to-day job will depend on the type of practice they work at, their colleagues, and their work preferences. Many radiologists in a private practice setting will read various studies outside of their subspecialty training. Still, an MSK radiologist may be asked to provide arthrography or MSK ultrasound services at outpatient centers. Academic MSK radiologists will typically focus heavily on their subspecialty, if not exclusively within. The job requirements of an academic MSK radiologist may include a variety of CT-, fluoroscopic-, and ultrasound-guided procedures, in addition to diagnostic imaging. MSK CT and MRI studies generally do not constitute a significant emergency and inpatient volume, but general and subspecialty call will depend on how the practice divides labor. Most MSK radiologists will be expected to competently read studies outside their subspecialty as a part of their call expectations.

References

1. National Resident Matching Program, Results and Data: 2024 Match® Results Statistics - Radiology. Statistics by Specialty: Musculoskeletal Radiology, Appointment Year 2025. National Resident Matching Program, Washington, DC. 2024.
2. Policies and Guidelines: 2024-25 SCARD Fellowship Embargo Guidelines. The Society of Chairs of Academic Radiology Departments (SCARD). Accessed March 2025. https://www.scardweb.org/policies.
3. Musculoskeletal Radiology Milestones. The Accreditation Council for Graduate Medical Education. Implementation Date: July 1, 2021; Second Revision: May 2021; First Revision: February 2014. Accessed March 2025. https://www.acgme.org/globalassets/pdfs/milestones/musculoskeletalradiologymilestones.pdf.
4. ACGME Program Requirements for Graduate Medical Education in Musculoskeletal Radiology. The Accreditation Council for Graduate Medical Education. ACGME-approved Focused Revision: February 7, 2022; effective July 1, 2022. Updated to include revised Common Program Requirements, effective July 1, 2023. Accessed March 2025. https://www.acgme.org/globalassets/pfassets/programrequirements/426_musculoskeletalradiology_2023.pdf.
5. Koval ML. Medscape Radiologist Compensation Report 2024: Bigger Checks, Yet Many Doctors Still See an Underpaid Profession. Published May 24, 2024. Accessed March 2025. https://www.medscape.com/slideshow/2024-compensation-radiologist-6017156.

Chapter 16
Neuroradiology/Interventional Neuroradiology

Kiran Talekar

Neuroradiology is a subspecialty of radiology, which focuses on diagnosing diseases and abnormalities of the brain, spine, and head and neck. Interventional neuroradiology focuses on various forms of vascular and nonvascular interventions for the brain, spine, and head and neck. Neuroradiologists undergo 1–2 years of neuroradiology fellowship training after a radiology residency. A few also pursue optional additional training in interventional neuroradiology or pediatric neuroradiology. Most programs offer a 1-year ACGME-accredited fellowship. A handful of programs may provide a second year, including more focused training on specific aspects such as vascular and nonvascular interventions, pediatric neuroradiology, head and neck radiology, etc.

Starting with the R1 (first year) of radiology residency, it is important to explore all radiology subspecialties. Radiology subspecialties can vary greatly in types of imaging modalities, cases, amount of patient interaction, number of procedures, amount of inpatient work, and, more importantly, future career prospects. It is important to develop an understanding of the benefits and drawbacks of each subspecialty. For example, radiology residents who pick neuroradiology have almost a 50–50 mix of inpatient and outpatient work during their fellowship year and in the future if they choose academia. They will use various imaging modalities, including magnetic resonance imaging (MRI), CT scan, fluoroscopy, and radiography. Overall, neuroradiology graduates are considered experts in MRI, the chief imaging modality in neuroradiology. Functional neuroradiology is an exciting and rapidly expanding part of neuroradiology. While historically, neuroradiology predominantly consisted of anatomic evaluation and diagnosis, new advances in functional neuroradiology allow physiologic and brain function studies such as brain mapping

K. Talekar (✉)
Thomas Jefferson University, Philadelphia, PA, USA
e-mail: kiran.talekar@jefferson.edu

© The Author(s), under exclusive license to Springer Nature
Switzerland AG 2025
J. Shames et al. (eds.), *A Radiologist's Path*,
https://doi.org/10.1007/978-3-031-86882-5_16

and white matter tractography. Functional neuroradiology is one of the fastest-growing fields for basic science and clinical translational research.

Neuroradiology graduates choose jobs in academia, community radiology, private practice, teleradiology, and emergency radiology in fairly equal numbers. In essence, neuroradiology graduates will have a wide variety of career options. An academic career is based on the three pillars: patient care, education, and research. It offers excellent opportunities for a more immersive neuroradiology practice, with a good balance of inpatient and outpatient work, including procedures. Academic neuroradiologists will also add value to patient care (beyond routine case readouts) by significantly contributing to clinical interdepartmental patient care conferences such as brain tumor boards, head and neck tumor boards, epilepsy conferences, etc. Research is a foundational pillar of academic radiology. Neuroradiologists have great opportunities to educate medical students, radiology, and other medical residents and fellows.

Neuroradiology graduates who choose community radiology or private practice typically spend 40–60% of their time reading neuroradiology cases. Community radiology practices and a growing number of private practices may have a small amount of inpatient work and interdepartmental patient care conference responsibilities. Neuroradiology graduates are also highly eligible for emergency radiology jobs, which offer the opportunity for shift work, which some prefer. Teleradiology is another career path with opportunities for remote work, which is becoming increasingly integrated into the other careers mentioned above.

If a radiology resident discovers that they are interested in pursuing a neuroradiology fellowship, there are several steps an applicant must complete to ensure a successful match. One fantastic resource to review is the ASNR (American Society of Neuroradiology) Fellowship Portal, which offers a general overview of the process, a list of national programs, and other helpful information for prospective applicants. It is important to research various programs, especially when looking for 2-year programs and more focused programs such as interventional neuroradiology programs. Like several other radiology subspecialties, the neuroradiology fellowship process utilizes the Match process. Diagnostic radiology residents will already be familiar with the Match process, as the NRMP (National Resident Matching Program) and ERAS (Electronic Residency Application Service) also manage the application process for diagnostic radiology during the fourth year of medical school. To complete a successful neuroradiology match, it will again be essential to register with the NRMP and ERAS.

It is fine and quite common to finish the first year of radiology residency and be unsure of which future fellowship to pick. Reaching out to mentors, speaking with department faculty, and discovering what kinds of studies you enjoy reading most are all worthwhile endeavors during the R1 year to help select fellowships. During R1 and continuing into the R2 year, finding a research project within neuroradiology can be beneficial. While not strictly required for a fellowship application, many institutions may favor applicants who showed interest in completing research during the selection process. While neuroradiology fellowship has a high baseline match rate, more desirable programs (due to location/education/etc.) can be quite selective. Demonstrating an interest in expanding and improving neuroradiology can be a desirable attribute.

By the end of the R2 year, an applicant should begin to identify their future letter of recommendation writers. Applicants will need three letters of recommendation: one from the applicant's program director and two from additional neuroradiology faculty. By the end of the R2 year, it is also important for applicants to begin to consider whether they would like to stay at their current institution or go elsewhere for a fellowship. This will come down to several personal and interpersonal factors, such as proximity to friends/family, educational and research opportunities, desire to stay at their current program/department, and opportunity to move to a new location.

At the start of the R3 year, neuroradiology applicants must register for ERAS in July. Supplemental documentation must be submitted during this process, including the three letters of recommendation, an applicant's curriculum vitae (CV), exam scores from the previously taken USMLE exams, personal statement, professional photo, medical school transcript, and medical school dean's letter. It is important to begin gathering this documentation, especially the letters of recommendation, in July of R3 year. The essential dates of the ERAS process will be posted on their website yearly, but the general overview is the following: ERAS applications are typically submitted by mid to late November, so completed letters of recommendation must be uploaded by then. In November of the R3 year, it is crucial to ensure that all required documentation is submitted at this time. By December, neuroradiology fellowships can view applications and start offering interview invitations, and applicants will be at a disadvantage if their application is not completed promptly.

With the online interview formats currently universally offered, applicants are interviewing at more and more programs unless limited to a geographic area. Programs typically interview 10–12 applicants for each fellowship position. However, as there are only 0.8 applicants per position (based on "Results and Data for the 2023" appointment year published by the Specialties Matching Service), this number may vary between institutions.

During this application process, it is also essential to register with the NRMP match during the R3 year, which typically opens in March. The essential dates will be posted yearly on the NRMP website. Typically, applicant ranking of programs they interviewed at starts in April of the R3 year, and the final ranking must be submitted by May. Match Day (when applicants discover whether and where they have matched) will occur in June.

Neuroradiology historically has a high match rate for prospective applicants. The match rates for neuroradiology are published yearly. Of the 261 applicants applying for neuroradiology in 2022, 95.6% matched the specialty. In the 2022 match, 90 available neuroradiology fellowship programs offered 305 available positions. Of these programs, 67% were filled completely, and 85.6% of neuroradiology positions nationwide were filled.

Neuroradiology is an extremely exciting subspecialty of radiology, which offers an immense variety of job prospects, the option of performing procedures (if desired), the ability to partake in cutting-edge research, and a daily workflow that is extremely interesting, challenging, and mentally stimulating. For more information, applicants are encouraged to view the ASNR fellowship portal.

Reference

1. Fellowship Portal - American Society of Neuroradiology. https://www.asnr.org/in-training-neuroradiologist/fellowship-portal/

Chapter 17
Nuclear Medicine Fellowship

Sophia R. O'Brien and Austin R. Pantel

In the United States, there are five Accreditation Council for Graduate Medical Education (ACGME) approved pathways for nuclear medicine (NM) training [1, 2]:

1. Diagnostic radiology (DR) residency (all DR trainees are exposed to NM during their general DR training and can read NM studies after graduation, but trainees do not receive a specific NM certification via this pathway).
2. Combined nuclear medicine-diagnostic radiology residency.
3. 16-month pathway (nuclear medicine fellowship integrated into diagnostic radiology residency)
4. Nuclear medicine fellowship (a one-year fellowship following DR residency).
5. Nuclear medicine residency (a completely separate residency from DR).

For discussion of combined nuclear medicine-diagnostic radiology residencies and nuclear medicine fellowships integrated into diagnostic radiology residency, please see Chap. 3 of this book.

The current chapter will focus on stand-alone nuclear medicine/radiology fellowship, a one-year fellowship after completion of a diagnostic radiology residency. Radiologists pursuing this pathway can obtain specialty certification in nuclear radiology (NR) from the American Board of Radiology or specialty certification in nuclear medicine (NM) from the American Board of Nuclear Medicine depending on specifics of their training program.

S. R. O'Brien (✉) · A. R. Pantel
Division of Nuclear Medicine Imaging and Therapy, Department of Radiology, University of Pennsylvania, Philadelphia, PA, USA
e-mail: Sophia.Obrien@pennmedicine.upenn.edu

J. Shames et al. (eds.), *A Radiologist's Path*,
https://doi.org/10.1007/978-3-031-86882-5_17

Application Timeline

Typically, radiology residents will begin thinking about fellowship in the spring of their R2 year with applications in the late fall/winter of their R3 year. Unlike some radiology fellowships, NM/NR fellowships do not participate in the NRMP Match process [3]. Some NM/NR fellowships follow Society of Chairs of Academic Radiology Department (SCARD) application guidelines [4]. For programs following SCARD embargo guidelines, applications may be accepted beginning in early November with interviews typically beginning in January or later (with exact dates defined by SCARD). Applicants have a grace period before they need to accept or decline any fellowship position offers. According to the 2023 SCARD embargo guidelines, after the grace period, applicants have only 1 day to accept or decline an offer [5]. Some NM/NR fellowship programs do not follow SCARD guidelines so may have a different timeline than above, and, notably, different amount of time given to an applicant before a decision on a fellowship spot offer must be made. The AMA FREIDA search engine (freida.ama-assn.org) is a great way to start looking at programs.

When Choosing a Nuclear Medicine Fellowship

There are many things to think about when choosing to which nuclear medicine fellowship(s) to apply. Like all medical training, location and proximity to family and friends should be considered. Additionally, your ideal job characteristic will influence the priority you place on certain aspects of fellowship training. Do you want to work in private practice, academics, a hybrid practice, or a VA? Do you want your job to include teaching, research, advocacy, and/or leadership roles? Do you want to look for a job in the same institution as your fellowship training or do you want to take your learning from fellowship to a different institution? There are no right or wrong answers, and no answer is set in stone, but these questions will help you work backward to determine the type and location desired for fellowship training.

When looking at the specifics of a nuclear medicine fellowship program, there are many questions to consider. How many fellows are accepted on average per year? Does the program tend to fill its slots (i.e., are there recent years with few or no fellows?). Does the program have other pathways, such as the 16-month integrated nuclear radiology fellowship and/or a combined NM-DR residency, and how do the different pathways align and interact? What specific educational curriculum is offered? What authorized user designations may be obtained following training?

NM Diagnostic Training

A strong NM fellowship should provide training and experience in adult general nuclear medicine and positron emission tomography (PET), pediatric general nuclear medicine and PET (at the same institution or via a collaborative agreement with a nearby children's hospital), nuclear cardiology, and radiopharmaceutical therapy. As new PET radiotracers receive FDA approval, strong programs will include these tracers in their everyday workflow. Current common adult PET radiotracers include 18F-FDG (still the workhorse of PET imaging), Cu-54- and Ga-68-DOTATATE imaging for neuroendocrine tumors, F-18- and Ga-68-PSMA imaging for prostate cancer, and 18F-FES for metastatic/recurrent estrogen receptor positive breast cancer. Pediatric imaging studies include both PET/CT and PET/MRI with 18F-FDG as well as many other radiotracers depending on an institution's historical experience, research interests, and patient population.

Radiopharmaceutical Therapy

Both NM and NR fellowships require classroom training and experience in administering radiopharmaceutical therapy including low and high doses of oral I-131 and a variety of parenteral radiopharmaceuticals [2]. The specific numbers required for each type of therapy vary pending which training exam (ABNM vs ABR) the trainee aims to take.

Current common IV radiopharmaceuticals include lutetium-177 DOTATATE ("Lutathera") for metastatic neuroendocrine tumor, Lu-177 PSMA ("Pluvicto") for metastatic prostate cancer, radium-223 ("Xofigo") for painful bone-dominant metastatic prostate cancer, and I-131 MIBG for advanced pheochromocytoma/paraganglioma in adults and neuroblastoma in children. Not all NM divisions will offer all therapies, and some may offer additional research therapies. Identifying the types of therapies offered and the volume of therapy patients seen by the division will give you insight into the patient populations you will be working with and your expected comfort with radiopharmaceutical therapy by the time of graduation.

Didactics

Well-established NM fellowship programs will have dedicated didactics for nuclear medicine fellows and often case conferences and journal club as well. The fellowship may also have teaching opportunities for fellows such as resident lecture, resident board review, NM fellow lecture/case conference, or even medical student teaching.

Fellow Responsibilities

NM and NR fellows may have nuclear medicine specific call duties on nights or weekends. Fellows may also be required to do general call or night float for the institution's radiology department. Moonlighting opportunities may be available.

Nuclear medicine physicians often lead radiology review of a multitude of tumor boards, but unlike other radiology specialties, NM/NR physicians can contribute to tumor boards as treating physicians for disease treated in NM therapy clinic. Fellows often prepare and present the tumor board imaging cases with mentorship by NM faculty. The specific tumor boards to which fellows will be exposed and the number of tumor boards fellows are expected to lead per week or per month will vary by fellowship.

Fellowships may provide academic time during which fellows can prepare for tumor boards and/or nuclear medicine clinic and work on their scholarly pursuits. The amount of academic time, if any, will vary by fellowship and sometimes by year pending the number of fellows in that year's cohort.

Other Considerations

Depending on your career interests, other considerations may include research opportunities (bench, translational, and clinical), leadership opportunities, and amount of mentorship/sponsorship provided by NM faculty.

Conclusion

Nuclear medicine is a dynamic and varied patient-facing field which is currently evolving at a rapid pace. New imaging radiotracers and therapy radiopharmaceuticals introduced in recent years are truly changing the field, and additional developments are likely right on the horizon. Nuclear medicine physicians provide diagnostic reads for a variety of nuclear imaging studies, serve as important consultants in multidisciplinary tumor boards, and function as the treating physician for multiple patient populations seeking radiopharmaceutical therapy. Your career goals will determine which of the factors described above are most important in your future NM/NR fellowship. Word of mouth is also a very important method of collecting information about a program—your residency institution's NM faculty can often help identify which NM/NR fellowship programs would be a good fit for you. Best of luck, you will be great!

References

1. Arevalo-Perez J, Paris M, Graham MM, Osborne JR. A perspective of the future of nuclear medicine training and certification. Semin Nucl Med. 2016;46(1):88–96.
2. American Board of Nuclear Medicine. Training Requirements for the ABNM Ceritfying Examination; 2023. https://www.abnm.org/exam/training-requirements/. Accessed 1 July 2023.
3. National Matchin Program. Radiology Fellowship Match; 2023. https://www.nrmp.org/fellowship-applicants/participating-fellowships/radiology-fellowship-match/. Accessed 1 July 2023.
4. Socity of Chairs of Academic Radiology Departments. 2023–24 SCARD Fellowship Embargo Guidelines; 2023. https://www.scardweb.org/policies. Accessed 1 July 2023. https://www.abnm.org/exam/training-requirements/
5. SAR, Society of Abdomial Radiology. SCARD Guidelines Agreement for Fellowship Program Directors; 2023. https://abdominalradiology.site-ym.com/page/SCARDagreement. Accessed 1 July 2023.

Chapter 18
Pediatric Radiology

Shashi Ranganath

Pediatric Radiology

One of the few subspecialties of radiology where it is possible to be formally sub-specialty boarded, pediatric radiology is focused on imaging children, from babies through adolescence. There is additional fetal imaging training in many fellowships, including prenatal ultrasound and fetal MRI, pediatric interventional radiology, neuroradiology, nuclear medicine, and other elective time, depending on interest/needed skill level.

Pediatric radiologists interpret most, if not all, imaging modalities and have specialized knowledge of pediatric patients' illnesses and medical conditions, many of which are unique to childhood and require an understanding of embryology and development. Collaborative relationships between pediatric radiologists and other pediatric subspecialists, such as pediatric urologists and orthopedic surgeons, are often solid, with close communication between caregivers to provide optimal care. Considerations such as a child's ability to cooperate with an examination, need for sedation/anesthesia, and radiation dose are all factors at the forefront of a pediatric radiologist's mind when determining the best imaging for a patient.

Further subspecialization within pediatric radiology is also an option, including pediatric neuroradiology, interventional radiology, fetal imaging, and nuclear medicine. Both academic and private or integrated care settings may offer the opportunity to practice pediatric radiology purely, though often nonacademic practices also include adult imaging interpretation.

S. Ranganath (✉)
Department of Diagnostic and Interventional Radiology, Mid-Atlantic Permanente Medical Group (MAPMG), Rockville, MD, USA
e-mail: shashi.h.ranganath@kp.org

J. Shames et al. (eds.), *A Radiologist's Path*,
https://doi.org/10.1007/978-3-031-86882-5_18

Chapter 19
Interventional Radiology Fellowship

Thea Moran

The Interventional Radiology "Fellowship" Versus Integrated IR Residency

The integrated radiology residency was discussed in Chap. 2; since medical students usually apply to this program, that chapter was presented with that audience in mind. However, much of Chap. 2 is also applicable to independent IR residency applicants. In Chap. 2, we discussed how to decide if IR is for you and we described how IR has evolved to a point where both the fund of knowledge and skill set required of an interventionalist is well past that which would be expected of a diagnostic radiologist. The American Board of Medical Specialties (ABMS) designated IR as a separate specialty in 2012, not as a subspecialty as it was previously. At present, there are two pathways for board-eligible IR training (Fig. 19.1). One pathway is through the integrated IR residency; this pathway is intended for medical students who have decided early that they want to practice IR. The other pathway is through an independent IR residency; this pathway may also be suitable for medical students who would like more diagnostic training than an integrated program would provide or for diagnostic radiology residents who decided later that they wanted to include IR in their practice. The independent IR residency functions like the traditional pathway (AKA IR fellowship, discontinued in 2020), except the independent IR residency requires 2 years of training and the previous fellowship required 1 year of training. An independent IR residency can be done with early specialization in IR (ESIR). This type of residency, essentially, is a hybrid of the integrated and independent IR residencies thus shaving 1 year off a subsequent independent IR residency. Since the independent IR residency functions similarly to the previous IR

T. Moran (✉)
MyriadMD Radiology Consulting, LLC, New Orleans, LA, USA
e-mail: tmoran@myriadmd.com

J. Shames et al. (eds.), *A Radiologist's Path*,
https://doi.org/10.1007/978-3-031-86882-5_19

Year	Traditional Pathway Offered thru 6/30/2020	Integrated IR Residency	Independent IR Residency Offered starting 7/1/2020	Independent IR Residency with ESIR Offered starting 7/1/2020
PGY-1	1 year of ACGME-accredited non-radiology clinical training (internship year)			
PGY-2	Diagnostic Radiology Residency	3 years of diagnostic radiology training	Diagnostic Radiology Residency	Diagnostic Radiology Residency with Early Specialization in Interventional Radiology (ESIR) included
PGY-3				
PGY-4				
PGY-5		2 years of IR training		
PGY-6	1 year of IR Fellowship		2 years of Independent IR Residency	1 year of Independent IR Residency
PGY-7	N/A	N/A		N/A
Total Years of Training	6	6	7	6

Fig. 19.1 Interventional radiology training pathways [1]. (Used with permission of the American Board of Radiology, current as of January 2024)

fellowship, it can only be done after completion of a diagnostic radiology residency. Despite it now being named interventional radiology residency, it is listed under fellowships in ERAS and NRMP and is discussed under the fellowship subcategory in this book. No attention will be given to international medical students or transfers from other programs in this chapter.

All ACGME- or RCPSC-accredited IR residencies will require an internship before starting IR training. There are requirements for your ACGME-accredited internship year which are the same as for diagnostic radiology [2]. Your medical school can direct you to the office that will have that information.

Applying to Programs

It is not just important to find an independent IR residency that will be a fit, but to find a diagnostic radiology residency that provides IR rotations (or ESIR training) that prepares you for an independent IR radiology residency. The Electronic Residency Application Service (ERAS) website gives the basic 411 on the available diagnostic and independent IR radiology residencies; more information on diagnostic radiology residencies can be found in Chap. 1. There are currently 94 independent IR residencies listed in ERAS [3]. While there are 94 independent IR residencies listed, not all residencies participate in ERAS. Applying for independent IR positions occurs during the third year for positions commencing immediately after diagnostic residency.

Independent IR residency applicants will need to specify whether they are applying as an ESIR candidate or a non-ESIR candidate. There are currently 170 diagnostic radiology programs with an ESIR designation listed on the SIR website [4]. An application will require the diagnostic radiology/ESIR program director to submit a standardized letter as part of your ERAS independent IR residency submission package to confirm that a resident applying to an independent IR residency has been accepted into an ACGME-approved ESIR curriculum. Clearly, no such letter is needed if you are a non-ESIR candidate [3].

After you have selected your program "short list," you then need to do your own research. I suggest you find out what each program considers important in an applicant and what the program accreditation status is (full accreditation, probation, etc.). Just because a program is listed somewhere, it does not mean it is ACGME-accredited or has not been sanctioned, so read the "fine print" and dig deep to make sure the program has full accreditation.

Information specific to independent IR residency applicants would be how hard a move would be if your diagnostic residency is far from your independent IR residency; you may want to weigh the quality of education in your two programs (if they are far from each other) against the annoyance of moving. If you are interested in ESIR, and since you will need to apply for that position during your diagnostic radiology residency application, see if you cannot be proactive and find out what the ESIR selection process is for whatever diagnostic radiology programs you are applying to; it may save you from applying to a diagnostic program that has a less advantageous ESIR selection process. Mentors are invaluable in deciphering information, generic and otherwise.

Register with ERAS after you've decided what independent IR residency you would like to apply to. Not all programs go through ERAS, but most do, and ERAS does streamline the process. Make well-thought-out selections because the application process can get expensive and overwhelming. Residents apply for the independent IR program through ERAS ACGME/RCPSC/UCNS Fellowship—December Cycle during PGY-4. The application process can be confusing so I would create a table/spreadsheet listing the programs you are applying to, what documentation is required (by ERAS and otherwise) from their applicants, and the ERAS/NRMP/institutional deadlines, with boxes to check off when something is complete. Things can come up with referees and other people you may have to rely on, so get started early. Currently, ERAS has a 2024 application timeline on its website [5]; be mindful that dates will change yearly, so check the website as per the year you're applying. Residents who would like to be considered for ESIR need to match into a diagnostic radiology residency that has an ACGME-approved ESIR designation. More details on how ERAS works are in Chap. 2.

Interviewing

Many of the suggestions in Chap. 2 on "Interviewing" are applicable here. Specific to independent IR residents, you will want to ask what your role would be at each program. Some programs will require you to assume the role of a junior attending (especially during your second year) and, if that is the case, then you are going to want to delve into specifically what that would entail (supervising diagnostic residents, lecturing, publishing, etc.). Other programs may go with the assumption that their incoming independent IR residents don't know anything so, their training approach is more instructional and supervisory. You will also want to ask how much "hands-on" experience can you expect to get (especially if you are at a program where you may be competing for cases with ESIR or integrated IR residents)? This is very important to know because hands-on experience is priceless!!!! For the ESIR candidates, it would be wise to ask, or get clarification, about each program's ESIR selection process during each of the diagnostic radiology interviews. What is very cool is that the NRMP has a Program Rating and Interview Scheduling Manager (PRISM®) that lets you track and rate programs during the application/interview process [6]. More on the NRMP in the next section.

The Match

NRMP is separate from ERAS. Independent IR residents participate in the NRMP Radiology Fellowship Match which requires a separate application and set of deadlines. There is a Match checklist on the website that can help stay organized [7]. There is also a Fellowship Match Calendar which gives a general idea of where the deadlines fall, but they will vary to year, so I would start checking the deadlines during the third year [8]. Match results come out in June for positions starting in July of the following year. There is no SOAP process for fellowship candidates, but a list of unmatched and matched programs that are only available to those who registered for the Match prior to the applicable Rank Order List Certification Deadline [9]. The registration fee(s) is/are the same as for the integrated radiology residency match. The rest is as per Chap. 2.

Rotation Specifications of Independent IR Residencies

The ACGME specifies that the resident is required to complete at least 23 months of IR or IR-related rotations; of the 23 months, at least 18 must be in the IR suite under the supervision of an interventional radiologist, and there must be 1 month of critical care training [10]. For ESIR candidates, you will be required to have 11 months of IR-related rotations where 8 months of these rotations occur in the IR section under the supervision of IR faculty during your final diagnostic radiology year. Also, during your final year, 1 month in an ICU rotation and a minimum of 500 image-guided procedures within the domain of IR are required

[11]. Residents are required to report cases they participate in through the ACGME case log mechanism [12].

Pathway to Initial Board Certification

Residents who are already board certified in diagnostic radiology only need to take the oral component of the IR/DR certifying examination [13]. An oral exam study guide is on the website [14]. If you did the ESIR year, then your board certification process is the same as that of an integrated resident.

Maintaining Active Board Certification AKA Maintenance of Certification (MOC)

Board eligibility begins immediately after residency and ends 6 years later or at board certification, whichever comes first. The American Board of Radiology grants every resident who passes both the qualifying and core exams and successfully completes an IR residency, IR/DR board certification. The Maintenance of Certification (MOC) process begins immediately after initial board certification. The MOC requirements are the same for all board-certified IR/DR physicians regardless of the pathway you took. MOC participation is mandatory for active board certification and active board certification keeps you marketable. MOC requirements/participation guidelines can be found on the ABR website [15].

References

1. Interventional Radiology. Initial Certification. Interventional Radiology Training Pathways. https://www.theabr.org/. Updated December 18, 2023. Accessed 13 Jan 2024.
2. ACGME Program Requirements for Graduate Medical Education in Diagnostic Radiology pp. 21–22. www.acgme.edu. July 1, 2022. Accessed 17 Jan 2024.
3. ERAS 2024 Participating Specialties and Programs. ACGME/RCPSC/UCNS Fellowship – December Cycle. Interventional Radiology – Independent. www.aamc.org/eras/. Updated June 8, 2022. Accessed 17 Jan 2024.
4. Society of Interventional Radiology. Early Specialization in Interventional Radiology. IR Training Option for Diagnostic Radiology Resident and Medical Students. Current Diagnostic Radiology Programs with an ACGME-approved ESIR Designation. https://www.sirweb.org/. Accessed 17 Jan 2024.
5. Electronic Residency Application System (ERAS) ERAS® 2024 Residency Timeline | Students & Residents. https://students-residents.aamc.org/eras-tools-and-worksheets-residency-applicants/2024-eras-residency-timeline. Accessed 13 Jan 2024.

6. The Match: Your Guide to Fellowship Matches: Interviews. https://www.nrmp.org/fellowship-applicants/. Accessed 17 Jan 2024.
7. The Match: You Guide to a Fellowship Matches. Fellowship Match Checklist. (www.nrmp.org). Updated April 2022. Accessed 17 Jan 2024.
8. The Match. Fellowship Participants Match Calendar. Master Calendar for all Fellowship Matches. www.nrmp.org. Accessed 17 Jan 2024.
9. The Match: Fellowship Applicants. What to Expect on Match Day. Unmatched Applicants. Common Questions. https://www.nrmp.org/fellowship-applicants/match-day/. Accessed 17 Jan 2024.
10. ACGME Program Requirements for Graduate Medical Education in Interventional Radiology, pp. 46–47. www.acgme.org. July 1, 2022. Accessed 15 Jan 2024.
11. ACGME Program Requirements for Graduate Medical Education in Interventional Radiology, p. 25. www.acgme.org July 1, 2022. Accessed 17 Jan 2024.
12. American College of Graduate Medical Education. Guidelines for Tracking Interventional Radiology Patient Care and Procedural Experiences. Review Committee for Radiology. https://www.acgme.org. Updated December 2017. Accessed 13 Jan 2024.
13. American Board of Radiology. Independent IR Residency. Initial Certification Overview. Passing the ABR Certifying Exam. https://www.theabr.org/. Accessed 17 Jan 2024.
14. American Board of Radiology. Initial Certification for Interventional Radiology. Studying for the IR/DR Certifying Exam. Oral Portion Study Guide. https://www.theabr.org/. Accessed 17 Jan 2024.
15. American Board of Radiology. Continuing Certification (MOC) Participation Guidelines. https://www.theabr.org/. Accessed 17 Jan 2024.

Part II
What to Expect After a Radiology Residency

Chapter 20
Your First Job Search and Career Tracks

Adam C. Zoga

Introduction

Congratulations, you've made it! You have dedicated years of your professional career and young life building a knowledge base, prepping for exams, learning where radiology fits in a health system, and working long hours, including nights, weekends, and holidays while sacrificing social life, family events, and monetary wealth to get to this position. You are no longer competing with hundreds of applicants for a few coveted positions, but instead, you are a desirable, valuable commodity throughout a vast array of healthcare organizations in all US geographic locations and many international [1]. You can design your own career, but ideally, you have already constructed several avenues toward your ideal job. Radiology is somewhat unique among medical specialties, in that post-training career choices should be considered and analyzed throughout residency, and the basic tenets of your post-training job should be established by the start of your final year of training, most frequently a subspecialty fellowship. There is a national and international shortage of radiologists, and the typical job of a radiologist is changing rapidly, with support and augmentation of imaging through artificial intelligence and the use of nonphysician radiology staff to perform and interpret some of the more basic exams [2–4]. You are in a position of strength, and early career options have never been more abundant.

To optimize your first postgraduate job in radiology, it is essential that you learn about the numerous options available for a career in radiology while completing your residency training. Unfortunately, this material is not always woven into radiology residency curricula, though many programs have initiated lecture series on the business of radiology. However, a wealth of information is available from the

A. C. Zoga (✉)
Thomas Jefferson University, Philadelphia, PA, USA
e-mail: adam.zoga@jefferson.edu

© The Author(s), under exclusive license to Springer Nature
Switzerland AG 2025
J. Shames et al. (eds.), *A Radiologist's Path*,
https://doi.org/10.1007/978-3-031-86882-5_20

attending radiologists you work with on a daily basis, as well as from any number of trade journals and online radiology business publications. Too often, as PGY-2 and PGY-3 residents are focused on learning how to communicate actionable findings or protocol an abdominal MRI or MRA of the brain, they miss out on the chance to learn life lessons on careers in radiology from their teaching mentors. Rising radiologists should push themselves to learn as much about the business and career opportunities in radiology during their first 2 years of residency as possible to leverage this knowledge base when choosing a subspecialty fellowship and, later, their first job as attending radiologists.

Corporate investment in radiology services, and subsequently in radiologists, is at an unprecedented level and shows no sign of reversal [5]. More than ever, residents and fellows considering their first job as an attending need to understand the radiology landscape. Residents should set aside time weekly to read the trade journal sites and include publications such as the Journal of the ACR and the RSNA Bulletin on their reading lists [6]. They should also find time during each rotation to ask their residency educators' opinions on where radiology is headed, what common job selection missteps they have seen, and what the optimal jobs in radiology will look like in 5 and 10 years [7, 8].

It is more than just salary. Burnout among radiologists is high, so each resident/fellow should consider how hard they wish to work, just how significant compensation is to them, and lifestyle considerations that might lead to a long, fulfilling career. Some higher-paying jobs require many evening or overnight shifts [9]. Others might include assignments across subspecialty areas that may drift far from a candidate's interests or training. Some jobs include shifts from home or flexible shifts, and vacation time varies widely. Private practice partnerships generally require a set period of time (track) to partnership and a financial investment in the practice (buy-in). One simple thing to factor into job selection is if the allotted number of vacation weeks includes the bookend weekends or if a week of vacation with the previous and following weekends actually counts for 9 days toward your time off quota. Continuing medical education (CME) and maintenance of certification (MOC) support is also widely variable. All radiologists are required to accrue CME for state licensure beginning 2 years after the conclusion of training, and it can be expensive. Many practices provide funding for CME activities, state licensure, and society membership. Without support, these fees can easily add up to $5000 per year or more. Other factors to consider include noncompete clauses and conflict of interest rules as delineated in any contract. It is shortsighted to think that bright, young radiologists can only make money being radiologists. If you develop an idea related to radiology and choose to bring it to market, it is important to know if your employer has the right to claim some ownership. Moonlighting can also be an issue, as some practices will not allow for radiology activities outside of the practice, but many others will [10].

The PGY-5 year is a great time to begin reviewing particular jobs and practices. However, it is important to remember that more desperate practices and health systems tend to post jobs and make offers earlier, while more stable practices, often offering the most desirable positions, may not post until within a year of the starting date. It is a buyer's market for radiologists in training, and there will almost always be multiple options. It is always nice to be flattered by an early job offer, but it is generally wise to consider multiple opportunities before signing a contract. In the current market, radiology residents can review the regional and national landscape and target a dream job with a stable employer in a desirable location.

Private Practice

Traditional private practices generally involve a corporation with ownership of some type of assets governed by a charter and practice leadership, including a president and a board of directors. Newly hired radiologists often receive a multiyear contract with pathways toward varying degrees of partnership or practice ownership. Criteria for advancement toward partnership can include time served, personal financial investment, productivity, and value to the practice. This type of practice is decreasing in prevalence across the USA, particularly in large metropolitan areas in the Northeast and on the West Coast. In the past 10 years, many solitary private practices have either sold to larger corporate entities, where the radiologists have less ownership and less autonomy but more centralized support [11]. Others have merged to form larger private practices, diluting equity and autonomy, or have simply sold to or been acquired by large health systems [12, 13]. There are still many traditional private practices in less populated regions of the USA, particularly in the Southeast and the Midwest. With a career path in private practice, contractual details are very important.

Taking a first job with a private practice should generally be considered a long-term commitment, in contrast to some of the other options discussed in this section. The path or track to partnership almost always takes time, and partners make higher and more sustainable incomes than non-partners. At the same time, investing in this type of commitment can lead to some of the highest long-term compensations for practicing radiologists, particularly if partnership is achieved and maintained. Subsequently, there are more variables to consider when considering a private practice job and reviewing a contract for such a position. Issues to consider include but are not limited to the following:

- Age of the practice and value to the community.
- Length and stability of hospital contracts.
- Assets and debts.
- Stability of radiologists in the practice.
- Size and support systems.
- External threats to the practice.
- Liability.
- Likelihood of achieving partnership and time to get there.
- Financial buy-in.

Many privately owned radiology practices in the USA have grown to become integral and appreciated service contributors to communities and health systems. Name recognition still holds value in radiology, and patients tend to show loyalty based on familiarity. Most private practices generate revenue from hospital contracts. Such contracts have life cycles and must be incrementally renewed. Short-term contracts are at greater risk of being lost to competition, such as expanding health systems and radiology management corporations. They also come with a risk of renegotiation, particularly if there is regional competition, which can devalue a radiology practice. These factors should be considered when evaluating a practice, as a significant change in hospital contracts can impact both compensation and your likelihood of achieving partnership.

Some private practices have invested in facilities, imaging equipment, and staff, while others use hospital or health system-owned equipment to provide services and rely almost fully on contracts and professional fees for revenue. A practice with tangible assets should be considered more stable than one without, but with the assets comes debt, and the debt/assets ratio should be considered when determining the stability of a practice. If you become partner, you become part owner of the assets and the debt. Certainly, a practice with ownership and sustained maintenance/replenishment of tangible assets is in a position of strength, particularly if they are set up to bill and collect technical revenues for outpatients or, even better, hospital-based patients.

The income disparity across radiologists within a private practice should also be considered. If multiple non-partner radiologists have joined and left the practice, this may be an indication of inequity. Larger groups tend to be more stable, but they may also include a lower percentage of radiologists achieving partnership. Other staffing considerations include teleradiology support and off-hour expectations. If the partners contribute little to off-hour coverage, overall radiologist staffing is generally less stable. Also, private practices should offer contracts that include strong liability programs with tail coverage. It is crucial that contracts be reviewed to ensure that you will not be left exposed or without tail coverage should you decide to leave before partnership.

No partnership is guaranteed until achieved even while investing into the practice. If the practice offers a five-year partnership track and there are regional threats to the practice, your likelihood of becoming a partner is not as strong as that of more stable practices without regional competition. If the private practice sells to a corporate or a health system before you become partner, you will not reap the benefits of the sale, though you may very well be offered a contract with the new owner, often without partnership opportunity. This is among the greatest drawbacks to considering joining a private radiology practice. You are absolutely at risk of not cashing in on a sale until you have at least some ownership, so the shorter the path to partnership, the better, and partnership pathways can often be negotiated.

Academic/Health System

Traditional academic radiology positions are also decreasing in prevalence as large health systems expand and generally employ a mixture of radiologist educators, community radiologists, and some true academic radiologists [14]. The near constant in this group is that radiologists do not own any part of the practice but are paid employees. These jobs can still be attractive, however, secondary to the strong benefits of employment and academic infrastructure [7].

The majority of radiologists who join an academic health system are partially compensated for teaching activities, both didactic and at the workstation, while a greater portion of the compensation stems from either the health system directly or a physician's practice plan. The latter part most frequently includes consideration of performance metrics, particularly clinical productivity. While variable, peer-reviewed publication and textbook authorship often play a small role in the compensation algorithm, and grant funding, while difficult in diagnostic radiology, can impact both compensation and clinical expectations. This type of job generally includes benefits related to lifestyle and work environment. Most radiologists enjoy teaching, and teaching comes with continuous, reciprocal, career-long learning. Teaching is not for everyone, however, and young radiologists joining a health system or academic medical center staff should be clear with their leadership how much they wish to contribute to radiology education. Often, contracts and job descriptions can be fitted to a young radiologist's wishes with a mutual objective of career advancement. There is always a balance, and while duties such as residency/fellowship program directorship can be rewarding and even glamorous, time dedicated to these jobs essential to our subspecialty is time away from clinical productivity. The practice compensation algorithm is key here, as being awarded 20% administrative time for educational/teaching endeavors does not necessarily mean that the comp plan will prorate you for these activities and reconcile your clinical expectations so that you are compensated in line with others generating more clinical RVUs (relative value units). An ideal compensation algorithm in a teaching practice employs an equation that compensates educators of all types fairly for their time, but building such an algorithm is no easy task.

There is a subset of radiology trainees who wish to dedicate their careers to academics. If you are one of them, get involved in grant writing early, as it is clearly a skill that improves with experience. There are vast opportunities for grant funding in radiology, including but not limited to artificial intelligence applications, oncologic imaging, functional neuroimaging, and image-guided therapeutic innovations [13]. However, writing your first grant is difficult, and based on my experience, grant writers are destined to accept a few failures before they get on a run of funded wins. Many academic centers in the USA support research, and building a career as a funded researcher is still possible, but the job search for such a candidate should really focus on academic centers with a research infrastructure, as a strong support staff plays a huge role in achieving success as a researcher.

As major health systems in the USA continue to expand, many of these systems tied to an academic hub have opened positions for community radiologists. These jobs tend to focus more on clinical productivity and less on teaching, but the ratio is widely variable. Often, community radiologists in a health system hold an academic rank, even if their teaching contribution is limited. This type of position in radiology has become both prevalent and popular in recent years, as health systems are beholden to providing quality imaging services, and radiologists get infrastructure support from the health system and the academic hub. CME and MOC play a role in every practicing radiologist's career, but these necessary exercises are easy to manage for radiologists affiliated with an academic hub. In fact, CME can become almost an afterthought if a community radiologist has access to the department and health system academic conferences and continued learning programs. Community radiology positions within a health system model can offer the opportunity to participate in teaching, a variably flexible schedule, and the security of working for a health system without the obligation to show academic productivity.

Further, health systems are increasingly recognizing the value of in-house radiology services and are becoming more creative in finding ways to keep this type of radiologist fulfilled and loyal to the health system. Throughout the USA, emergency departments order their greatest volume of imaging studies from early-midafternoon through the evening, often 3:00–11:00pm, but radiology staffing is most robust from a period more like 8:00am–4:30pm. This is an issue every health system that operates emergency medicine services wrestles with, but it is also an opportunity for younger radiologists to select work times that best suit their lifestyles while cashing in on the needs of the health system, either through increased compensation or shift flexibility and frequency. Many health systems allow for radiologists to perform emergency radiology shifts from home, another perk for many radiologists with families.

Career mentorship is more frequently available and practiced in groups with an academic hub, and mentorship can play a vital role in continued career growth and job satisfaction. Benefits are generally strong, including health system-supported retirement programs, dependent tuition scholarship programs, and family medical leave compensation for major life events. Full-time radiologists should make enough income to generate wealth, and health system retirement programs are often conservative but allow the program owner to manage as much as they like. At mid-career ages, many radiologists have children in college, and tuition reimbursement programs can be a major perk.

In contrast to private practice, taking a job with a health system does not need to be considered a long-term commitment. Most academic and health system positions include a modest obligation period should you decide to move on to another position, often in the range of 6 months. However, more and more health systems and practices are including restricted covenants or "noncompetes" in contracts, limiting employee migration to regional competing practices without financial penalty.

Corporates

Radiology practices have been hot targets for acquisition by wealthy venture capital/private equity firms for at least 10 years, and there are too many variations of corporate structure to review in this format [12]. One of the more common formats is when an established radiology private practice sells some or all of its assets to a firm for a price distributed to the practice shareholders. With this transaction, radiologists, particularly the partners, lose autonomy in exchange for the payout. There have been both success stories and failures after this type of deal, but once completed, there is no going back. In some cases, the radiologists have maintained control of practice management, while in others, the radiologists immediately become employees, governed by a corporate management structure and answering to a board of directors. There are many tracks for radiologists to gain shares or equity in the company, but none will reach the level of ownership that radiologists can attain with a private practice. One of the first tenets learned in any business school curriculum is "the primary objective of the board of directors is to maximize profits for the shareholders." Any radiologist taking a job with a corporate, non-radiologist owned firm must accept this simple fact, as management and board of directors' decisions should not be expected to primarily favor the radiologists, the practice, the hospitals, or the patients. They will favor the shareholders.

Still, there are many strong opportunities for radiologists within these corporate structures. Revenues for radiologists with strong clinical productivity are generally high, and radiologists can often build their job in an a La Carte sort of fashion, working harder and more frequently when they want and taking more time away from work when desired. Corporate entities managing radiology services are often large and frequently offer great infrastructure to help radiologists attain and maintain multiple state medical licenses and credentialing across multiple practices, but again, structures and offerings are widely variable. Many radiology private practices in the USA have sold to private equity corporations only to be spun off to health systems within a few years, so the radiologists themselves have three distinct employers over a short period of time. Some of the more successful corporations offering radiology services have woven in the radiologist-driven practice management infrastructure that made the private practice successful enough to be a target for corporate acquisition, but still the board of directors ultimately answers to the shareholders. In other scenarios, multiple private practice radiology groups have merged to become a larger, stronger corporation with the radiologists comprising a majority in equity ownership, but these radiologist-owned corporate practices still migrate toward the typical infrastructure of a for-profit corporation, with decisions in the best interest of the shareholders. The idea of part ownership in this type of large practice provides some reassurance to the radiologists that the company will act in their best interests, but individual radiologist ownership is significantly diluted when compared with a smaller private practice.

Particulars of each corporate job vary, and benefits offered should be thoroughly reviewed prior to signing a contract. Look for the employer to contribute to a retirement fund and ask about programs supporting family growth and dependent education.

There are many opportunities for early career radiologists to earn a strong income and seize opportunities in business by joining a large corporation, but significant ownership in the practice should not be the driving factor in choosing such a job, as it can be considered a longshot.

Teleradiology

Fully remote jobs have been on the market for more than 20 years and continue to grow their footprint in diagnostic radiology. Teleradiology positions maximize radiologist opportunities for flexible shifts and work-life balance, as there are emergency, inpatient, and outpatient imaging studies requiring interpretation somewhere at all hours of the day or week. For instance, practices and health systems in the Eastern USA often employ radiologists located in the Western continental USA or Hawaii to read off hours studies during the daytime in Western time zones. In recent years, numerous teleradiology groups have emerged, some radiologist owned and some corporate owned or supported by venture capital. Some teleradiology groups focus on one or two subspecialties, and some hire diagnostic radiologists in all subspecialty fields to provide full service to hospitals and health systems.

Teleradiology jobs are widely variable, and any applicant should take care to learn the expectations, potential for flexibility, and compensation structure before signing a contract. Per-click payment structures are popular with radiologists, but the work expectation remains a significant variable. An expectation that includes a large volume of studies with each shift, particularly with a per-click compensation system, can lead to radiologist burnout, while a small number of shifts or a less-than-desired number of cases to read can lead to disappointing compensation [11]. There is also a psychological element to working from home daily, and many radiologists with teleradiology jobs ultimately find a space to work outside the home, at least some days. However, these jobs remain very popular both with young radiologists who have family considerations and with older radiologists who no longer want to commute daily. Hospitals and emergency departments are often busiest in the afternoons and early evenings, so there are many teleradiology and health system jobs available that allow radiologists to spend time with family early in the day if they work into the evening.

While full teleradiology companies generally offer jobs that are 100% offsite, both health systems and private practices are more likely to offer jobs that include both onsite and offsite shifts. For candidates interested in part-time or full teleradiology careers, the options are numerous, and there are opportunities within all of the practice types reviewed previously.

Military

The US Armed Forces support a robust system of hospitals and outpatient health centers internationally, including diagnostic and interventional radiology. Many of my colleagues through the years attended medical school with a Health Professions scholarship through the US Army, Navy, or Air Force. Such a scholarship eases or eliminates the burden of medical school debt but comes with an obligation to the particular branch of the Armed Forces. I attended medical school on a US Navy Health Professions Scholarship, which covered medical school tuition and provided a stipend for living expenses throughout medical school. For this, I owed a year of service in the US Navy for each year of medical school funded. With such a program, candidates can complete internship, residency, and fellowship programs within the sponsoring branch of service or can apply for a deferral to complete training in a civilian program. Residency and fellowship training years, whether in uniform or civilian, do not count toward a service obligation, but years in training in uniform do count toward retirement, which many health professionals use as a foundational building block for late-career goals and retirement.

Attending radiologist jobs in the US Military can be subspecialized or general and can be at military facilities both within the USA and abroad. Many US Armed Forces medical facilities support state-of-the-art, cutting-edge radiology departments and some house radiology training programs and academic productivity. A career as a US military radiologist can be fulfilling and fiscally rewarding, but a military career essentially always includes relocation and the possibility of deployment to active military operations. Some radiologists who choose to serve in the US Military subsequently choose to remain in the service in the Reserve Corps after completing their obligation. This path offers a chance at achieving a US Armed Forces retirement but also includes the possibility of being called to Temporary Active Duty and subsequent disruption of the radiologists' civilian career, an issue that is more likely to be impactful on a radiologist in private practice and more likely to be accepted for a radiologist working for a health system. Another federal option for civilian radiologists is employment with the Veterans Administration Medical Center network. Clinical expectations in this setting tend to be lower, and compensation is good with federal employee benefits and pension as well as student debt relief programs.

Benefits for US Armed service members and their families are outstanding, and a radiology career in the US Military can absolutely support one's goals of early retirement or of moving to part-time work mid-career.

References

1. Konstantinidis K. The shortage of radiographers: a global crisis in healthcare. J Med Imaging Radiat Sci. 2024;55(4):101333.

2. Huisman M, Ranschaert E, Parker W, Mastrodicasa D, Koci M, Pinto de Santos D, et al. An international survey on AI in radiology in 1,041 radiologists and radiology residents part 1: fear of replacement, knowledge, and attitude. Eur Radiol. 2021;31:7058–66.
3. Wichmann JL, Willemink MJ, De Cecco CN. Artificial intelligence and machine learning in radiology: current state and considerations for routine clinical implementation. Investig Radiol. 2020;55(9):619–27.
4. Rawson JV, Smetherman D, Rubin E. Short-term strategies for augmenting the national radiologist workforce. Am J Roentgenol. 2024;222(6):e2430920.
5. Fleishon HB, Vijayasarathi A, Pyatt R, Schoppe K, Rosenthal SA, Silva E III. White paper: corporatization in radiology. J Am Coll Radiol. 2019;16(10):1364–74.
6. Scott-Blagrove J, Tharmalingham H, Obaro AE. Promoting equity of opportunity in radiology & oncology through mentorship and advocacy. Clin Radiol. 2022;77(4):239–43.
7. Khaja MS, Contrella BN, Wilkins LR, Pyne R, Majdalany BS, Rajebi R, et al. Issues most pressing to early-career interventional radiologists: results of a descriptive survey. Acad Radiol. 2022;29(11):1730–8.
8. Ortiz DA, Muroff LR, Vijayasarathi A. Early-career radiologists' perceptions of national corporations in radiology. J Am Coll Radiol. 2020;17(3):349–54.
9. Chen M, Gholamrezanezhad A. Burnout in radiology. Acad Radiol. 2023;30(6):1031–2.
10. Blythe JA, Flores EJ, Succi MD. Justice and innovation in radiology. J Am Coll Radiol. 2023;20(7):667–70.
11. Santavicca S, Hughes DR, Fleishon HB, Lexa F, Rubin E, Rosenkrantz AB, Duszak R Jr. Radiologist-practice separation: recent trends and characteristics. J Am Coll Radiol. 2021;18(4):580–9.
12. Hardy SM, Lexa FJ, Bruno MA. Potential implications of current corporate strategy for the US radiology industry. J Am Coll Radiol. 2020;17(3):361–4.
13. Lopez J. Private equity backed radiology considerations for the radiology trainee. Curr Probl Diagn Radiol. 2021;50(4):469–71.
14. Kikano EG, Ramaiya NH. Mentorship in academic radiology: a review from a trainee's perspective – radiology in training. Radiology. 2022;303(1):E17–9.

Chapter 21
Integrated Health Care Delivery Systems

Shashi Ranganath, Wilbur Chang, and Ainsley MacLean

Integrated Healthcare Delivery Systems

Although often when people think about career tracks, they most commonly refer to academics and private practice, another equally appealing option for radiologists is the integrated healthcare delivery system. What do we mean by this? Integrated healthcare delivery means that patients pay an annual fee to a health insurance provider which covers all services and that the health insurance provider owns and operates all the buildings and equipment in which the patient receives care. There are then physicians employed by the practice who provide care for patients within this system, and these physicians work in a salaried model. There is no direct incentive for physicians to do more surgeries, scans, or tests, and there is no incentive for the health insurance system to either. Overall, the healthcare delivery system, the physicians, and, most importantly, the patients benefit when patients are healthy, so everyone works toward this common goal. Kaiser Permanente and the Permanente Medical Groups are the most well-known example of this model and employ nearly 750 radiologists nationally. However, Geisinger is another example, among many others.

The radiologists who apply and interview with this model are often interested in practicing in a model where the patient and quality are the absolute epicenters. We hear stories of radiologists in the traditional fee-for-service payment model where spine surgeons are told to go into every little detail at every level, hoping this might generate more referrals. Since we all know that back surgery is rarely the cure for lower back pain, this is the opposite of a patient-centered approach to care. In an

S. Ranganath (✉) · W. Chang · A. MacLean
Department of Diagnostic and Interventional Radiology, Mid-Atlantic Permanente Medical Group (MAPMG), Rockville, MD, USA
e-mail: shashi.h.ranganath@kp.org

J. Shames et al. (eds.), *A Radiologist's Path*,
https://doi.org/10.1007/978-3-031-86882-5_21

integrated healthcare delivery system, standardized reporting is the guiding beacon, and less is often more.

Another advantage of being a part of an integrated healthcare delivery system is that communication between providers is transparent and facilitated. We all know how difficult it can be to interpret a complex radiologic examination when no information is given regarding indication and history, so readily available clinical data, including laboratory values, and ease of discussion between providers help improve and expedite care in an integrated health system. In addition, since all imaging stays within one care system, patients who receive an initial diagnosis within the system have postprocedural imaging as well, with pathology and laboratory reports easily accessible, and this contributes not only to longitudinal learning and pathology follow-up but professional satisfaction.

Chapter 22
Applications

Anne Kathryn Misiura

Introduction

Congratulations! You've done it! You've graduated (hopefully for the last time) and are now on to the next-last step!

You hopefully haven't graduated yet, because you should start looking for a job while still in training. In the current market, you might do this nearly 2 years before your anticipated start date. Fortunately, the world is currently your oyster, and instead of selling yourself to an institution, institutions will sell themselves to you.

Preparation/CV

Hopefully, you're reading this very early in your training and can take my advice sooner rather than later. You should be constantly updating your CV. Whenever you give a presentation or have a case report published, (call your mom and then) update your CV. This way, you will never forget to add something and will never need to take more than a few minutes fine-tuning before sending it off at someone's request during training.

However, you must trim the fat before sending this essential document out for jobs. Take a critical look at the ends of all your sections. My future employer does not need to know that I was on the planning committee for the turkey trot my first year of med school or that I volunteered in the gift shop at a hospital during undergrad. (I kept that I was vice president of the Pi Chapter of the Alpha Chi Sigma professional chemistry fraternity during my undergraduate years (Shout out to all

A. K. Misiura (✉)
Department of Radiology, Thomas Jefferson University Hospital, Philadelphia, PA, USA
e-mail: anne.misiura@jefferson.edu

© The Author(s), under exclusive license to Springer Nature Switzerland AG 2025
J. Shames et al. (eds.), *A Radiologist's Path*,
https://doi.org/10.1007/978-3-031-86882-5_22

my fellow AXE brothers. Yours in the double bond). I think it's good to have a few of these experiences still listed because it makes you look human! If you're having trouble with the selective reduction of your CV, ask one of your mentors to look it over for suggestions.

I'll caveat this advice by saying that if your CV is slimmer, you should focus on beefing it up instead.

You'll also need references. Your mentors should undoubtedly be on this short-list. Reach out to your letter writers from your fellowship applications. Your favorite attendings, even if you're applying to your current training institution and elsewhere, will be happy to be a reference for all applications. Nobody expects you to apply to just one job.

Cover Letter

This is not a personal statement. This concise summary summarizes who you are and what you're looking for. Introduce yourself, explain your situation, detail what job type you're seeking, and outline your career goals. That's it—no flowery statements or "This one time..." stories. If you're "cold emailing" for a job (not directly responding to an open position), cover letters are essentially what you're writing in the body of your email. If specifically requested by a job advertisement to send a cover letter with your CV, format it as a formal letter. Do not make this long (between 250 and 400 words suffices). Do an internet search for examples. This is easy to write and should not be a stressful exercise.

Applying

This should go without saying, but please keep track of where you're sending off applications, including the contact information for where it's going, any login information needed if it's an application site, the date you sent it, and any other relevant details. Don't overextend yourself. I'd argue that sending out ten applications at once is probably not a great idea, as you're juggling too much communication. I think it's wiser to apply to a couple of your top picks first and give it a few days to weeks to hear back.

Follow-Up

Be patient. Respond to interview offers promptly. Your training program will give you ample interview time, as they want you to succeed. If you haven't heard back from an institution you've applied to, follow up with them to inquire if they've received it. Waiting about 2 weeks for a response is reasonable. If you've accepted a job, it's good form to let other places know that, too. Nobody wants their time wasted. Being courteous will also keep the doors open to potential future employers. You never know when you'll need those opportunities.

Chapter 23
Where to Look for a Job

Thea Moran

You have finished your training and are ready to venture into the big wide world as an attending radiologist. Job well done! Now, you have to find your first job. This can seem daunting, but it is okay when you break it down into three steps:

1. What kind of practice do you *think* you want?
2. Where do you *think* you want to live?
3. Where do you look for a job?

1. What Kind of Practice Do You *Think* You Want?

There are two primary kinds of practice: private and academic. Teleradiology is commonly used in both practice types, at least partially. Both job types have their pros and their cons. Private practice options are either employed or have partnership tracks. Traditionally, practices have comprised physicians who provide clinical services to a community in either an inpatient or outpatient setting; hospitals contract directly with physician groups to provide services to their inpatients, and referring physicians send their patients directly to outpatient centers. Both vary in their volume, modalities provided, and culture, but there has been a trend to outpatient opportunities having fewer credentialling hurdles compared with inpatient. There are opportunities to work for corporate entities in either facility type, which is becoming more common.

Corporate doctors can feel a conflict of interest because the businesspeople can hire (and fire) with minimal influence from a medically trained intermediary (such as the head of a practice) to mediate. The important thing (whether it is traditional or employed practice) is to find a practice with similar priorities to yourself. One of my favorite workplaces has been with a corporation that owns outpatient imaging

T. Moran (✉)
MyriadMD Radiology Consulting, LLC, New Orleans, LA, USA
e-mail: tmoran@myriadmd.com

© The Author(s), under exclusive license to Springer Nature Switzerland AG 2025
J. Shames et al. (eds.), *A Radiologist's Path*,
https://doi.org/10.1007/978-3-031-86882-5_23

facilities throughout the country (and many of my coworkers there felt the same way). It could be frustrating because sometimes the left hand did not know what the right hand was doing (the company was so big), but there were plenty of helpful nonphysician and physician colleagues you could call on if there were any questions.

Academic practices are what you are most familiar with. These practices are affiliated with medical schools where you will be expected to provide clinical care, teach, and publish. Academic practices come in a variety of shapes and sizes. It is a common misconception that private practice is more fiscal minded than educational practice, but don't be fooled. Money makes the world go around, and academic medicine is no exception, regardless of their apparent lofty pursuits. The rise of the corporate model in educational practices has made the fiscal nature of academic medicine.

2. Where Do You *Think* You Want to Live?

Only honest self-examination can answer this question, and the questions you ask yourself will be specific to you. What part of the country do you want to live in? What kind of weather do you prefer? Do you like living in urban or rural locations? What would the commute be like if you like working in urban areas but want to avoid living in the city (and visa versa)? Do you have specific extracurricular activities that would exclude some parts of the country (good luck finding ski resorts in Florida)? Of course, with the above questions, your family status will determine their needs and preferences. These are just a few possible questions to get you started, but by all means, add more questions as you see fit.

3. Where Do You Look for a Job?

There are three main ways that people find jobs: job listings, headhunters/recruiters, and word of mouth.

Most major radiology societies have job sites where you can post as a job seeker or employer. The career centers at the American College of Radiology [1], the American Roentgen Ray Society [2], and Career Connect at the Radiological Society of North America [3] list jobs for all radiology positions and are widely used. Major subspecialty societies also post jobs on their websites; these sites are preferred if you are looking for a subspecialty practice. Many websites are free to look at and apply. Society journals also have job listing sections, so ask your department or go to the institution library for their most recent edition (the internet is probably more accessible, though). However, these job postings have a downside. Sometimes the listing needs to be updated, and sometimes, it is a job that was posted as a matter of policy. (i.e., the job poster already knows whom they want to hire, but the institution policy states that the opportunity needs to be publicly posted).

Headhunters/recruiters are people who do the job searching for you; you give them your filters then they find the job and present it to you. They may post your availability on a website and/or use their contacts (and they often have plenty) to find a suitable job. They can operate independently or work for a company. Make sure you work with a reliable recruiter/company. It is routine for headhunters to receive a finder's fee when they place a job seeker. Subpar recruiters/companies are a dime a dozen, and it can be troublesome if they send you someplace that is not a match. Ask people who have used recruiters and, if they have, who they recommend. Good recruiters will have been around a long time and have built up good word of mouth; if you cannot find a recommendation, go for a recruiter with a long track record.

Along a similar train of thought: locum tenens. Locum work can be temporary or temporary to permanent (an on-the-job interview, if you will). Some people like to go directly to the employer to contract for this kind of work, but I would not recommend it unless you know the client very well or there is a vested interest for the client not to take advantage of you. While your take-home pay may not be as much, the locum company knows the going rate for your services, sets up the contracts, and can act as an intermediary should there be "creative differences" between you and the client. Locum companies also have legal departments that cover your malpractice and will get involved should the client not want to pay. Solid recruiters are invaluable in these circumstances because they will steer you clear of a risky client, even if the client is listed with the company. Being responsive and helpful to a good recruiter's queries will help build relationships with these recruiters, who will likely work harder for you. Recruiter information aside, locum work provides opportunities to see different parts of the country and how other practices operate with varying case mixes. The pay is good, and travel and lodging are paid, but benefits are rarely included. Any job (but especially locum) can be daunting for a new graduate. Let your recruiter know that you are a recent graduate, and hopefully, they will be able to steer you toward a user-friendly environment. The National Association of Locum Tenens Organizations (NALTO) [4] has a directory listing its locum company members, but it is not exhaustive.

Word of mouth is my all-time personal favorite way to look for a job. There is no need to go to job sites applying for jobs that may or may not be available, and there are no middlemen. Networking is crucial to word of mouth. Networking may be a four-letter word for bookworms working alone in darkened rooms daily, but it is not that bad if approached with the right attitude. Networking is best viewed as making "new friends." Making plenty of friends who, in turn, have plenty of friends will put you in a great position to find a job by word of mouth. Always be yourself when meeting people; there are tons of practices, each with its quirks and preferences, and you are bound to find somewhere that is a fit. And keep doing the networking after you secure a job because practices can be sold and departments restructured. Situations conducive to in-person networking would be society, department, hospital, or city meetings. Finding a mentor and publishing with faculty within or outside your department (or geography) are also ways to network. Networking can occur remotely via social media. Social media platforms often have groups where people of similar interests discuss, and share, points of interest. You would be amazed at the number of, and different kinds of, opportunities that come up in these groups (Rad Chicks on Facebook is my favorite—an excellent forum for sharing information with a great group of lady radiologists). Doximity and ResearchGate are other social media platforms.

In a nutshell, that is how to find your first job. If there are a few jobs you find interesting, keep a spreadsheet where you can keep track of each practice's name, contact information, and details about each practice. Don't be afraid to reach out if you have not heard from them. And lastly, you may have noticed that at the beginning of the chapter, I said, "Practice types you *think* you want" or "places where you *think* you want to live." Sometimes, you have to try different situations before finding what works for you, and there is no harm. I wouldn't do this too much or too frequently, though, lest you appear like a poor bet on future applications.

References

1. American College of Radiology Career Center. https://www.jobs/acr.org. Accessed March 26, 2025.
2. American Roentgen Ray Society Career Center. https://www.arrs.org/jobs. Accessed March 26, 2025.
3. RSNA Career Connect. https://www.rsna.org/membership//career-and-professionalism/career-connect. Accessed March 26, 2025.
4. NALTO Agency Members. https://www.nalto.org/members/agency/. Accessed March 26, 2025.

Chapter 24
Interview Process

Anne Kathryn Misiura

It's time to prepare for your first (real radiology) job interview. The big difference from your earlier interview experiences for medical school, residency, and fellowship is that the institution is trying to sell itself to you. Don't get me wrong; you should have your best foot forward and make a good impression. They want to hire someone who'll fit in and be a great radiologist, but the balance has shifted, and you're not solely at the mercy of an admissions committee.

Give your training program ample warning of the time off needed for the interview. They must and will accommodate you. Some programs may offer two-day interviews and should let you know ahead of time if you're being taken to dinner the night before the interview day so that you can plan your travels. It is acceptable to ask if your spouse/partner is expected/invited to your interview dinner. Most programs/practices will cover your travel and lodging. If not booked for you, keep your receipts to submit for reimbursement.

Make sure your suit/professional attire fits at least a month beforehand. You don't want that packing day surprise.

Dress professionally. Arrive early to account for traffic. Be kind to everyone you encounter.

At this point, you've already identified the position as something you're interested in, but you will and should have many questions for the interviewers. In no particular order, here are some topics to get you thinking:

Staffing—coverage, work locations, nighthawk service, "on call," physician turnover, moonlighting opportunities.
Workflow—PACS, IT support, reading lists, productivity expectations, productivity measurement, peer review system.

A. K. Misiura (✉)
Department of Radiology, Thomas Jefferson University Hospital, Philadelphia, PA, USA
e-mail: anne.misiura@jefferson.edu

© The Author(s), under exclusive license to Springer Nature
Switzerland AG 2025
J. Shames et al. (eds.), *A Radiologist's Path*,
https://doi.org/10.1007/978-3-031-86882-5_24

Work volume—breakdown of cases, average daily RVUs, the complexity of cases, subspecialty preferences, procedures.

Electronic medical record and integration.

Dictation software.

Communication—stat result workflow, reading room assistants, protocoling.

Academia—resident/fellow schedules, academic time, research expectations.

Private practice—buy-in, partnership track, group structure, group ownership of imaging centers.

Technologists—skill set, turnover.

Support staff—skill set, turnover.

Hospital system stability and administration turnover.

Conference participation.

Salary, productivity bonuses, raises.

Vacation/CME/personal time, availability, and request process.

Malpractice insurance coverage.

Retirement plan.

Insurance plan.

CME stipend, business expenses.

Home workstations.

It would be best if you were observing the dynamics and behaviors in the practice. How new are the facilities? How eager are partners/staff to talk with you? How open are they with their answers? If you're interviewing solely with administration/chairs/chiefs and not meeting other radiologists, ask them why. No program/practice should be hiding its staff from you.

Picture yourself here in 3 years. Are you happy if nothing has changed? Is there something lacking now that you can ask about the potential for change in the future?

Be ready to answer questions you should have asked yourself before applying:

What kind of position are you looking for?

Which procedures are you comfortable with or willing to learn?

What kinds of studies are you willing to or not willing to read?

Where do you see yourself in one year? Five years? Ten years?

Fortunately or unfortunately, many radiologists will not stay at their first job for their entire careers. Until you have real work experience, it can be difficult to know what to ask about and prioritize in looking for the perfect position.

As of April 2025, there are 2,057 job postings on the ACR career board [1]. As I've mentioned previously, the world is currently your oyster. Don't settle, and get what you've earned.

Reference

1. Radiology jobs – American College of Radiology Career Center [Internet]. [cited 2023Feb25]. Available from: https://jobs.acr.org/

Chapter 25
Contract Negotiation and Legal Aspect of Contracts

Hamid R. Latifi

Introduction

So, you have finished your postgraduate training, completed your interviews at your desired jobs, and been offered a position with a radiology group. They send you an offer letter, also known as a "letter of intent," detailing the basics of the job, but later you receive the legally binding long document called the "Employment Agreement" or "Physician Contract." You need at least a basic knowledge of contract provisions, legal terminology, and the significance of your legal obligations. Furthermore, it would be best if you were comfortable with some negotiating skills to make you happy at your first job and check the most boxes on your wish list of salary and benefits that you desire to get from your future employer.

This chapter briefly overviews necessary contract negotiation and legal understanding of an employment contract. These two topics are closely linked since, most of the time, you have received several oral promises at your interview, but now comes the actual written agreement, which may contain all or most of the verbal commitments, and many more obligations spelled out for both parties to the agreement —you as the prospective employee and the entity that will be hiring you as the employer.

H. R. Latifi (✉)
Department of Radiology, Baylor University Medical Center, Dallas, TX, USA
e-mail: hlatifi@americanrad.com

© The Author(s), under exclusive license to Springer Nature   129
Switzerland AG 2025
J. Shames et al. (eds.), *A Radiologist's Path*,
https://doi.org/10.1007/978-3-031-86882-5_25

Finding a Physician Contract Attorney

Most people at your stage of life have seen only a few legal contracts; for instance, lease agreements for the apartments you have rented in the past, and a purchase or lease agreement for your automobile. And let's be honest, how many people read those long, tedious documents filled with confusing legalese? However, now the situation is different, and the stakes are much greater. Therefore, it is crucial to have an experienced attorney review your contract and advise you before signing your first contract. The best way to find an attorney to review your employment contract is by referral from someone who has had a positive experience with that attorney. Otherwise, you should seek an attorney specializing in healthcare law and with experience reviewing physician contracts. Preferably, you would want to seek legal counsel from an attorney with expertise in radiology contracts, and may even be your subspecialty in radiology. Alternatively, you can seek an employment law attorney with experience with physician contracts.

A detailed discussion of contract law is beyond the scope of this book, but you should be familiar with at least two aspects of contract law, which I will oversimplify here. First, a tenet of contract law is that contracts are written such that their provisions favor the party who drafted them. Therefore, since you are handed a contract drafted by well-paid and experienced attorneys who work for your employer, you can assume the terms will not favor you in a contract dispute. As you will see in the following sections, you can negotiate to make some terms more favorable, but only some provisions will be negotiable. Second, you can assume that if something is not explicitly written in the contract, it will not be honored by a court of law.

Therefore, if you care about a specific oral promise made to you during the interview or afterward, in an informal letter, email, or phone conversation, you want to ensure it is written in sufficient detail in the final written contract to be legally binding.

Contract Negotiation

Generally, radiologists' job options include working in a private practice radiology group, hospital or multispecialty group, academic center, or a hybrid model (e.g., a private practice group that trains radiology residents and fellows). Solo practitioners, or small groups, who own their imaging centers, are becoming extinct in almost all large cities in the United States. Over the past few decades, the trend has been toward "mega groups" with dozens, if not hundreds, of radiologists. Within the private practice paradigm, most new graduates will pursue a partnership track position to become a "shareholder" in the group after a certain length of time, and share in the group's profits and other benefits. However, other options in a private practice group may include working as a non-partnership-track full-time or part-time employee, or an independent contractor. Regardless of the setting or position, you will inevitably face the challenge of negotiating your best terms after reviewing the employment contract.

In my opinion, contract negotiation, at its essence, boils down to a straightforward question that you must ask yourself: "How badly do I want this job?" The answer to this question will determine the framework of your negotiation. If your geographic location is restricted to a large metroplex because of family or other personal reasons, you likely will have limited leverage when negotiating the terms of your contract. For instance, if an elite group in Manhattan has offered you a job, which is the job you want to have because you love New York City, you and your spouse have family ties to the area, you have just become a new parent, and being close to family is crucial, then you have little room for negotiation and may have to sacrifice much of your wish list to get the job. However, suppose you have no geographic restrictions, family ties, or other personal preferences and get an offer as the only interventional radiologist in a small town in the middle of Nebraska. In that case, you most likely will have the upper hand at the negotiation table. These two extreme scenarios illustrate the dependence of the negotiating power on the answer I posed at the beginning of this paragraph. Suppose you must have a job in a limited geographic area saturated with radiologists. In that case, your negotiating power is much less than if your choice of ideal living place, climate, population density, and amenities is less restricted or not restricted at all. The following sections in this chapter will review the essential components of the contract that need scrutiny and the utmost attention to prevent future regrets and potential legal problems.

Important Contract Sections

Salary

Your starting salary as a new graduate is integral to your consideration for accepting a particular job. Still, it must be considered together with the "benefits" package to truly understand the entire value of your compensation. The salary is also likely one of the most negotiable terms in your contract. How do you know what to expect and what is a fair salary? Again, the answer is tied to your desire for the particular job. Suppose you love the position offered to you, and you think you must have it. In that case, you can still negotiate, but you may have to settle for less than your salary goal to gain the intangible benefits of working in a particular group at a specific geographic location or academic institution. In almost all cases, the salary is usually discussed during the interview or shortly afterward in verbal communication or the offer letter. There are online resources to look for median physician salaries, but the best idea for a fair wage can be obtained by asking a colleague in your subspecialty. Of course, this is a sensitive topic that most people are uncomfortable disclosing. Still, you will undoubtedly have mentors at your training program willing to help you understand the salary expectations in your geographic area. Suppose you have been to multiple interviews and discussed salaries with different groups. In that case, you will have a good idea about the salary range offered in your target area.

Benefits

Universally, your employer will offer certain benefits; if these basic benefits are not offered, run the other way and do not look back! Some of the most common benefits are discussed below, but the list does not encompass all the benefits and the many variations of the same benefits.

Malpractice Insurance

Your group should pay for your malpractice insurance. The only exception is if you are working as an independent contractor, in which case you should expect few benefits, if any. For most of you starting your careers, you will be a full-time or part-time employee—likely in a partnership track—and should expect your employer to pay for your malpractice coverage. There are two types of medical malpractice insurance coverage: "occurrence" and "claims-made" coverage. The distinction between these policies becomes very important if you change jobs, which according to Santavicca et al., more than 40% of radiologists did within 4 years examined in their study [1].

An occurrence policy covers incidents while the insurance policy is active, regardless of when a claim is reported to the carrier. For instance, if an occurrence policy covered you while you worked for a radiology group from 2012 until 2016, at which time you resigned and joined another group, and if you are sued in 2018 for an incident that happened in 2014, then you are still covered by your previous employer's insurance policy. In contrast, a claims-based policy provides coverage if the incident took place *and* the policy was in the effect at the time a claim is filed. For instance, in the same scenario as above, when you worked for a group from 2012 until 2016, you will not be protected if a claim is filed in 2018 for an incident that occurred in 2014! However, if the same claim was filed before you left your previous group in 2016, then you are protected. Most groups will offer claims-based policies to cover their physicians and advanced practice providers, which means you have to know and understand the type of coverage you have if you ever decide to change jobs and leave your group.

Fortunately, there is a solution to protect you after your claims-based policy is no longer active, and the answer is "tail coverage." This is where the details of who will provide the tail coverage and how much it will cost become crucial, and must be precisely detailed in your employment contract. There are many approaches to tail coverage, varying from one employer to another. Moreover, this is another provision that you may want to negotiate. Many groups will require the employee who is leaving the group to pay for their tail coverage—which, by the way, is not cheap—but some may pay that expense if you have been employed with that group for a certain number of years, or many other variations on the theme. Of course, if you are lucky enough to be protected by an occurrence policy, you will not need to purchase tail coverage if you change jobs.

Health Insurance

Your group should pay for your primary health insurance, although there may be an additional charge for your spouse and children. They may offer you dental and vision coverage at an additional out-of-pocket cost.

Other Benefits

Your employment contract should outline vacation, sick, and holiday time, as well as details of the call and weekend coverage, and if there is extra compensation for call and weekend coverage, how such payment is calculated, and possibly an allusion to whether that compensation amount is different for new hires, "junior partners," and full partners. Almost all private practice radiology groups and academic institutions will pay for your state's medical license dues and Drug Enforcement Administration (DEA) permit and renewal fees, as well as provide time and reimburse expenses for continuing medical education (CME) activities required to maintain active licensure and participate in the maintenance of certification (MOC) program of the American Board of Radiology (ABR).

Many groups will offer long-term disability insurance, and some may even provide short-term disability insurance. Many groups may offer nominal life insurance policies, with options to buy additional coverage at your own expense, typically offered at rates lower than an individual policy for the same amount of coverage in the outside market. However, beware that most disability and life insurance policies are valid only while employed by your group, and do not carry over if you leave the group. So, although the coverage may be offered at a lower price, you may want to look into purchasing a separate life insurance policy—and disability insurance policy—outside of your employer-offered policy, which you then own regardless of where you work.

Many groups offer moving expenses to help ease the financial burden of moving from wherever you are finishing your residency or fellowship to another part of the country where your new job is located. Although uncommon, some employers may offer a sign-on bonus if you join the group.

Partnership Provisions

If you are joining a private practice group that offers a partnership track, make sure that there are clear written terms in the contract that explain how you can achieve a full partnership. These terms include the length of time you must work at a fixed salary before you are eligible to become a full partner, which will typically allow you to share in the group's profits by various bonus structure models, and give you voting power in your group's governance. Once you are a full partner, you likely will be eligible to participate in various committees or become a director on the group's board. Many groups will require a "buy-in" before you can become a full partner. This is a certain amount of money you must pay to the group to purchase the privilege of becoming a partner. The group may require you to pay the amount in one lump sum or installments over a specified time. When you leave the group— by resignation, termination, retirement, or death—you will receive the same amount back from the group as a "buy-out."

Restrictive Covenant

As a healthcare attorney and practicing radiologist, I believe this is one of the most critical provisions in your employment contract. These provisions, more commonly known as noncompete clauses, are intended to protect an employer's interests by restricting a departing physician's ability to practice medicine within a designated geographic area for a specified period after termination of employment [2]. Such restrictive covenants are illegal in some states, such as Massachusetts, Delaware, and Colorado. Still, they are common and have been upheld in most states, when deemed reasonable in duration and geographic scope [3]. The "reasonability" of duration and geographic area is often case-specific. These restrictions must be reasonably tailored to protect the employer's legitimate business interests without unduly infringing upon the physician's livelihood. For instance, an unreasonable and overbroad restriction may eliminate a physician's ability to practice in an entire state upon departure from the current employment. Factors that affect the determination of the enforceability of noncompete clauses include, but are not limited to, population density of the area, radiologist shortage in the area, and the nature of the physician's termination. The rise of teleradiology in many group practices across the country has challenged the enforceability of these restrictions and created a debate about the usefulness of noncompete clauses in general [3]. For instance, when a large radiology practice interprets radiologic studies for numerous imaging centers and hospitals across a large metropolitan area or an entire state, what is "reasonable" geographic restriction without essentially forcing the departing radiologist to move to a different city or a different state altogether for the duration of the noncompete clause?

Considering the opposing interests of employer and employee physician in the scope of noncompete clauses, this is an area where you want to negotiate as much as possible to find common ground with your prospective employer, such that they are protected from you opening an imaging center across the street from one of their centers. Still, at the same time, you will not be required to uproot your entire family and move to a different state to continue earning a living.

Another restrictive covenant included in almost all contracts is the non-solicitation clause. In contrast to noncompete clauses, most non-solicitation clauses are fair and necessary to protect the employer's interests in its proprietary and non-proprietary assets, including their nonphysician employees and allied healthcare professionals. In simple terms, these clauses prohibit the leaving physician employee from soliciting and "stealing" the employer's nonphysician employees by encouraging them to leave their current employment and join the departing physician at a different facility, especially if that would be a competing facility.

Termination

All employment contracts should clearly state the conditions for termination and the duties of each party in the event of termination. Almost all of the radiology contracts in the United States, with minor exceptions, are "at will," which means that both parties to the contract may terminate the agreement at any time with or without cause, as long as the employer's reason for removing the employee is not illegal. The difference between contracts lies in the details of what is considered "cause" for the employer to terminate the agreement, and the notice requirements. Generally, a longer notice time favors the employer, and a shorter one favors the employee. For instance, if you want to leave your current group and accept another job, neither you nor your new employer will likely be happy to be required to wait for 6 months after you hand your resignation letter to your current employer before you can start your new position. Generally, a common compromise is a 60–90-day notice requirement, so that the employer has an opportunity to fill your position. Of course, if the termination is for cause and the situation jeopardizes the employer's vital interests or patient safety, the termination may be immediate, as it may be necessary to have you pack your stuff and leave the premises as soon as possible!

Miscellaneous

Most physician contracts place restrictions on your outside activities, especially if those activities interfere with your work schedule or competency to perform your duties on the job, or if those activities in some way compete with the employer's interests.

Concluding Remarks

This chapter serves as a general introduction to physician contracts. It motivates you to carefully read and understand your entire employment contract, not only for your first postgraduate job but also for any other positions you may consider in the future. The contract provisions outlined in this chapter are not meant to be all-inclusive, but a sampling of the more essential requirements in a physician contract and their meanings. The sections are intended to provoke you to think about the possible implications of what you are signing, not only when you accept a particular job but also long-term expectations at your current job, and future consequences if and when you ever depart your current job.

Disclaimer The author of this chapter has contributed to this publication solely in his personal capacity. All views and opinions expressed herein are the author's own and do not reflect the positions of his respective employers or affiliates, including, but not limited to, Latifi Law, PLLC, Avicenna Consulting, PLLC, Baylor University Medical Center, and their respective affiliates (collectively, the "employer entities"), and should not be interpreted as legal advice. You should not act or rely upon this information without seeking advice from a lawyer, in each case licensed in your jurisdiction, as applicable. Neither the author nor any of the employer entities are responsible for any errors or omissions in the content of this publication or any damages arising from the use of this publication or any information provided herein, in whole or in part, in any format, under any circumstances.

References

1. Santavicca S, Hughes DR, Fleishon HB, Lexa F, Rubin E, Rosesnkrantz AB, Duszak R Jr. J Am Coll Radiol. 2021;18:580–9.
2. Wiley MB, Polsinelli VE, Asheld BA. Restrictive covenants. J Am Coll Radiol. 2015;12:645–7.
3. Mezrich JL, Siegel EL. Noncompete clauses: a contract provision that has exhausted its usefulness? J Am Coll Radiol. 2014;11:145–52.

Chapter 26
Financial Aspect of Contracts (Salary and Bonus)

Shashi Ranganath

While we get outstanding radiology training during our residencies and fellowships, unfortunately, many of us need more education on financial considerations when looking for our first job out of training. Earning potential is multifactorial, and many factors should be considered. Salary is the primary consideration, but it is essential to know how this relates to daily expected workload, remote/onsite/hybrid shifts, off-hours shifts, weekend shifts, weeks of vacation, and cost of living. Will you read burnout-level volumes of cases and must offset some of your "vacations" to recover? Is a weekend shift a Friday night through Monday morning or an 8- or 12-h shift on a Saturday or Sunday?

Total compensation is a more accurate descriptor than salary, and benefits, including malpractice coverage, 401k contributions, healthcare/insurance coverage, license/fee reimbursement, and retirement, are all essential items to consider. Leadership opportunities or developing skills in your current position, which may lead to more lucrative jobs within or outside of your practice, also come into play. Equal compensation based on transparent metrics and advancement opportunities are critical considerations for long-term happiness at a job. With rising radiology volumes, there are often opportunities to "moonlight" internally or pick up extra shifts, and depending on how much additional work you are interested in, there can be a considerable increase in income.

Often, salary and significant benefits are not flexibly negotiated, but it is worth asking about signing bonuses (though read the fine print!), forgivable loans or loan payoffs, and moving stipends as these smaller incentives can add up and are easier

S. Ranganath (✉)
Department of Diagnostic and Interventional Radiology, Mid-Atlantic Permanente Medical Group (MAPMG), Rockville, MD, USA
e-mail: shashi.h.ranganath@kp.org

to inquire about, depending on the current job market state. Smaller items to ask about that may add up over the long term are childcare, gym, or electronics discounts that many larger hospitals or integrated healthcare/larger systems have in place.

Chapter 27
Gender Inequality in Compensation

Gilda Boroumand and Kristina Nowitzki

Spend time speaking with women in radiology. You will find that many (perhaps most) of us have experienced some iteration of the same story: lower compensation for the same work. This is true in both private practice and academics. Some of these stories are decades old, but many are from the last few years. We are told that contracts are nonnegotiable and identical for all employed radiologists, only to find out later that our contemporaneous male colleagues were offered higher starting salaries, special sign-on bonuses, better relocation expense reimbursement, shorter paths to partnership, or all of the above. Even when we try to negotiate for what we know has been offered to our male colleagues, we are met with a metaphorical pat on the head. "Oh, you would like XYZ benefit, like we offered the male radiologist straight out of fellowship? Sorry, that's only for critical recruits." Or "That extra degree you want us to sponsor for you through the medical school? That would take you away from your family… you should consider a weekend course that will get you a nice certificate at the end." Insert exploding head emoji.

These stories are not few and far between, and the evidence is not just anecdotal. In the Physician Compensation Report published by Doximity in 2021, women in medicine still earn about 28% less than their male counterparts [1]. The numbers specific to radiology are similar. In 2018, male radiologists responding to the Doximity survey earned an average of $442,000, while women earned $349,000, a difference of 21% [2]. This made radiology the specialty with the fourth highest wage gap that year. In the following years, radiology managed to stay out of the top 5, but almost all specialties had wage gaps of over 10%.

Maybe you have seen the published studies describing no gender pay gap in radiology [3]. While these seem reassuring, they were based on data collected from a small subset of public academic centers required to release salary data publicly.

G. Boroumand (✉) · K. Nowitzki
Department of Radiology, Norwalk Hospital, Norwalk, CT, USA
e-mail: kristina.nowitzki@nuvancehealth.org; gilda.boroumand@nuvancehealth.org

© The Author(s), under exclusive license to Springer Nature Switzerland AG 2025
J. Shames et al. (eds.), *A Radiologist's Path*,
https://doi.org/10.1007/978-3-031-86882-5_27

The Doximity data suggest the same does not hold for private academic institutions or private practices. The studies could also not fully capture incentive components of pay, such as bonuses or other income sources, which add to a physician's overall revenue.

The basis for the gender wage gap is often a subject of heated discussion, and commonly perceived factors such as specialty selection or individual productivity cannot fully explain it. While social and workplace dynamics lead to a greater percentage of female radiologists choosing to work part-time, this also does not account for the Doximity data, which are based on full-time positions (defined as working at least 40 h per week). A thoughtful article by Pandit et al. outlined several social and systemic factors that may be contributing to the wage gap in radiology [4]. For instance, medicine traditionally demands "overwork" of its physicians and prizes those ideal workers who can work long hours and be on call 24/7. As the authors point out, this "overwork" environment "rests on a social foundation that is itself highly gendered: employees who work long hours can only do so with support from others, usually from women, who shoulder more household and unpaid work obligations." In this environment, employers and employees are socialized to perceive those working part-time or having family obligations as less productive or uncommitted, with subsequent pay structures constructed to reward and incentivize overwork.

Moreover, the definition of "productivity" may be based on inequities. Many practices compensate radiologists based on the number of RVUs they generate. Yet, in many departments, the necessary non-RVU-generating work, such as teaching trainees, interacting with patients, and assisting technologists, is shouldered disproportionately by female radiologists. In certain practices, leaders have recognized their role in perpetuating pay discrepancies and restructured their departmental compensation schemes [5]. But this change is not yet far-reaching. So, what is a female radiologist to do in the meantime?

When searching for a job, your best defense against inequity is networking. This will give you insight into compensation structures, work-life balance, volume expectations, practice culture, etc. Speak to as many radiologists as you can and gather whatever information they are willing to share. Social media is a good resource for unfiltered information, though you may want to take most of the information there with a grain of salt. Physician groups on social media post spreadsheets with anonymous, self-reported physician salaries, including information on gender, practice type, full vs. part-time, location, etc. Though not validated, this will give you an idea of what is possible in your part of the country. Know that *every* job offer is negotiable, and that men frequently negotiate when women don't. Ask your male friends (including those outside medicine) how they would negotiate; you may be surprised by what they ask for. It is a tightrope to balance, as women who negotiate can be perceived as annoying and overbearing, while men who negotiate are perceived as tactical and ambitious. But, as more women expect and ask for fair compensation, culture and expectations will continue to improve.

Advocating for yourself doesn't end once you sign an employment contract. You may become aware of certain inequities—for example, in the assignment of vacation and call shifts or in the doling out of bonus or after-hours compensation—only after you start your job. You may find that you will consistently have to ask for what you want, which may be things that your male colleagues already ask for and get or even get without asking. You may notice that you are perceived as uncommitted because you don't buy into the "overwork" demands of medicine and instead strive for work-life balance.

The gender pay gap in medicine is stubbornly persistent, so women must continue pointing out the inequities in our practices and seeking systematic change. But we can't simply wait for system changes to take place. On a practical level, we have to be willing to advocate for ourselves throughout the span of our careers. We must articulate the value we bring to our practices and expect—indeed, demand—to be fairly compensated for it.

References

1. Doximity. Doximity 2021 Physician compensation report. 2021. https://assets.doxcdn.com/image/upload/pdfs/compensation-report-2021.pdf. Accessed 1 Mar 2023.
2. Doximity. Doximity 2019 Physician compensation report. 2019. https://assets.doxcdn.com/image/upload/pdfs/physician-compensation-report-2019.pdf. Accessed 1 Mar 2023.
3. Kapoor N, Blumenthal DM, Smith SE, et al. Sex differences in radiologist salary in U.S. Public medical schools. AJR Am J Roentgenol. 2017;209(5):953–8.
4. Pandit R, Minton LE, Smith EN, et al. Equal pay for equal work in radiology: expired excuses and solutions for change – clinical. Imaging. 2022;83:93–8.
5. Edwards M. Improving pay equity. American College of Radiology; 2021. https://www.acr.org/Practice-Management-Quality-Informatics/Imaging-3/Case-Studies/Strategic-Planning/Improving-Pay-Equity. Accessed 8 Feb 2023.

Chapter 28
Applying for Privileges/Licensure

Kristina Nowitzki

Licensing

Each US physician must obtain a medical license issued by the US state or jurisdiction where they plan to practice. There is no reciprocity. So, if you plan on working in multiple states due to living close to state lines or practicing telemedicine, more than one state license may be needed. To try and simplify this process, an Interstate Medical Licensure Compact was formed in 2015. So far, over 33 states and territories have participated in this compact, reducing the application burden, not the overall cost. To learn more information and see a map of participating states, visit https://imlcc.org.

Every state has different procedures and requirements for licensure. A significant first step in the process is to look at the website for your condition and gather information on their needs and required documents. The individual website can be found using a simple internet search, or links can be found on the Federation of State Medical Board website (https://fsmb.org/contact-a-state-medical-board).

In general, each state will ask for verification of education and graduate training and documentation of passage of a national licensure examination (USMLE or CMLEX-US). You will also be asked to submit information affecting your ability to practice medicine, including health status, criminal convictions, and malpractice settlements or judgments. Many boards conduct criminal background checks. It is best to be forthcoming with any derogatory information. In most states, making a false statement on an application will result in denial of licensure or restrictions.

Licensure usually requires renewal every 1–2 years to ensure you maintain acceptable standards. There is almost always a CME requirement which may include some state-specific required training (e.g., medical ethics, pain

K. Nowitzki (✉)
Specialty Imaging, Danbury, CT, USA

© The Author(s), under exclusive license to Springer Nature Switzerland AG 2025
J. Shames et al. (eds.), *A Radiologist's Path*,
https://doi.org/10.1007/978-3-031-86882-5_28

management, and prescription of opioids). So, be sure to keep up to date on your individual state's requirements.

The entire process of obtaining a medical license takes, on average, 2–3 months, with overall longer processing times for international medical graduates. Several states, including Alaska, California, and Texas, have longer average times for obtaining licensure. While you must have a medical license before completing hospital credentialing, it is best to get started on both as soon as possible.

Credentialing

Credentialing is the process healthcare organizations use to onboard new physicians and ensure their patients are in skilled hands. It involves three linked but separate processes: credentialing, privileging, and enrollment.

It all starts with credentialing, extensive verification, and physician qualifications approval. This is a mandate for hospitals and other healthcare organizations set forth by regulatory and accreditation organizations, including the National Committee for Quality Assurance (NCQA) and The Joint Commission (TJC). In addition to having an active medical license, a hospital's credentialing board wants to ensure you have the appropriate training to perform services for your patients. This step will include an application specific to the hospital or organization and requesting several supporting documents. It is crucial to fill out the application as complete as possible. Also, communicate well with your group's credentialing coordinator and the organization's credentialing office. This will alert you to any missing information or a delay in receiving the requested documents.

Specific documents to gather in preparation for this step include:

- Education, training, and board status (certification or eligibility)
- Work and medical staff history
- Any clinical privilege history
- Names and emails of peer references
- Malpractice insurance carriers and any claims history
- Federal, state, and professional licenses and registrations
- Explanation for any 30-day gap in education, training, or work history

The next step is privileging, in which the organization authorizes you to perform specific services. This is a requirement set by the Centers for Medicare and Medicaid Services (CMS). The credentialing office will request which procedures you would like to obtain privileges for, often as part of the abovementioned application. It is best to include as many procedures/services as possible within your scope, as it is usually harder to add these privileges later.

The last step is enrollment which allows you to bill for services and get paid. You must apply for participation in each relevant health insurance network as a medical provider, including national payers such as Medicaid and Medicare and major commercial payers. The process will usually be done on your behalf by the appropriate administrative office using all the documentation gathered above. However, plenty of specific forms will require your information and signature.

Final Thoughts

The licensure and credentialing process is easy but often long and tedious. Be sure to start earlier than you think, as this can be the rate-limiting step in getting to work. Be sure to keep organized. Your future self will thank you; chances are you will need to repeat the process sometime in your career.

Chapter 29
Moving

Anne Kathryn Misiura

When I was a young, bright-eyed first-year attending, my husband and I packed up our life, our epileptic cat, and our four-week-old child and drove over 1000 miles to a new home and new job. I don't recommend the experience. I had not yet completed a year at my first job before moving on to the second. I am a part of that statistic. But as someone who's moved 14 times since I left for my first year of undergraduate education, this was old news, albeit the first time with a small child.

Moving sucks. But you're a planner if you're reading this book, and planning makes all the difference.

Let's make this easy. There are several circumstances to consider:

Short moves can be done in a day or two or stretched out over a more extended period for convenience. If you have help, great. If not, hire some help. It won't break the bank, and the convenience can't be beaten. You're more in direct control of things with short moves. You can supervise packing, loading, and unloading with movers and follow the truck so you always know where your stuff is. If you can manage most of your belongings, but there's a very heavy couch, and your old apartment is a three-floor walk-up, hire movers by the hour to handle this. These are the most straightforward moves and should cause little to no stress.

Single moves are just you and some stuff. In these cases, it's usually easiest to buy your friends a case of beer to help load/unload and drive the truck yourself or with a buddy. Make it a fun road trip. Pay for your buddy's flight back home. Use this time to do some sightseeing if it's a more protracted move.

Long moves require a several-day drive or flight. Here is where expenses can add up. Estimating costs at each level would be best to determine your budget. What do you hire out, if anything? Packing? Loading? Transport? Storage? Unloading? Are you driving or flying? Look into insurance for all of these steps if you do hire

A. K. Misiura (✉)
Department of Radiology, Thomas Jefferson University Hospital, Philadelphia, PA, USA
e-mail: anne.misiura@jefferson.edu

© The Author(s), under exclusive license to Springer Nature   147
Switzerland AG 2025
J. Shames et al. (eds.), *A Radiologist's Path*,
https://doi.org/10.1007/978-3-031-86882-5_29

out. Are you comfortable with your stuff potentially being MIA for a few days? It's not unusual for movers to load multiple people's belongings onto trucks for long hauls across the country. Longer hauls equal a higher risk of damage and loss. They probably won't be working on a strict time frame. A coresident and his family of five drove for two days to get to their new home. Their stuff was delayed a week behind them. So, prepare for this scenario. Where will you sleep when you get there? When my partner moved to a new state, he ordered a BedInABox to arrive before he did. These foam mattresses have gotten pretty great. Whatever you decide, have a backup plan to the backup plan and be flexible.

Family moves are multiple people and probably a lot more stuff. Outsource as much as possible. Pack up some suitcases as if you're going on vacation for a week or two and hire a company or someone you know to drive your things for you. Taking your time is probably more important than saving a couple of hundred bucks in any step here. If you can, use this time to do a little vacationing, mainly if you're waiting on a professional truck to deliver your life. Go to Disney, the Grand Canyon, or Niagara Falls. The more you can do to enjoy this time, the less stressed you'll feel.

Whatever your circumstance, prepare for something to get lost or broken. Remember, everything is replaceable except you and your humans/pets.

Now, about packing. Use this opportunity to take stock of your stuff. Declutter. Throw out. Channel your inner Marie Kondo. You do not need to ship your USMLE books across the country. Trust me; you don't need them anymore. Similarly, those cans of refried beans do not need to be boxed up. Donate to your local food bank. Those suits or dresses you wore in high school or college will not (read: should not) be worn again. Find a clothing donation center before you go. Purge what can be purged.

Determine the expense of moving your old mattress across the country versus buying a new one. Consider this with every large furniture item you own. If you're feeling savvy, list things for sale online. Donate furniture to incoming residents or fellows.

My final advice is always to pack a bag as if you're going out of town, even if you're only moving across the city. Take your suitcase and fill it with the essentials for a day or more. This should include your pajamas, toothbrush, essential toiletries, medications, wallet, and probably your most valuable small possessions (jewelry, birth certificates, social security card, passport, etc.). This goes with you and never on your moving truck. This way, you don't have to dig through boxes and bags to prepare for bed.

It's also beneficial to have a survival kit. I pack a bag including toilet paper, paper towels, cleaning products, disposable cups/plates/cutlery, hand soap, dish soap, and essential tools (screwdriver/hammer/wrench). Anything you may need initially while unpacking that you don't want to search boxes for should go in your survival kit.

I also try to ensure that the vacuum goes on the truck last in case you get a messy surprise when you arrive at your new home. Unloading into a clean house or apartment is much nicer than the alternative. Does your mother-in-law want to help? Send her to the new place to clean before you get there. Delegate tasks that don't involve someone else packing or unpacking your underwear.

Enjoy the process and the new adventure. Go ahead and order a pizza on your first night. You've earned it.

Further Reading

https://www.jacksonphysiciansearch.com/white-papers/early-career-physician-recruiting-retention-playbook/

Chapter 30
Other Practice Considerations

Shashi Ranganath

Additional Practice Considerations

When exploring practices after residency or fellowship, it is essential to note that the scope and practice of radiology are highly diverse, and there are many considerations that residents and fellows may need to learn are important or which to ask about when looking at jobs after training. When investigating a practice, the best way to understand the workflow and culture specifics is to speak with radiologists in the group, especially of various tenures. Is the newest hire, who has been there less than one year, happy? What about the radiologist about to retire who has been in the practice for 25 years? The mid-career radiologist is often the most valuable fount of information as they have been there for enough time to know the ins and outs of the practice. It is very reassuring if they plan to stay until retirement for many more years.

Culture is hard to assess until one is more engaged in the practice, but it is essential to ask about that, though much depends on you and what type of person you are. While no job is perfect, finding the best fit for what you are looking for and ensuring expectations align with your new practice is essential. Understand the volume and pace of reading expectations, if it is a hybrid practice or purely onsite vs. remote, and what the PACS/IT and technologist support is like. Assess whether a practice is dynamic or tends to stay more stagnant and hesitates to embrace change. Are they exploring innovative technologies in workflow facilitation, such as AI (artificial intelligence)? Are volumes being assessed and rotations updated based on data?

One of the most important considerations is how radiology quality concerns are addressed. At some point, all of us will miss a significant finding in our career, but

S. Ranganath (✉)
Department of Diagnostic and Interventional Radiology, Mid-Atlantic Permanente Medical Group (MAPMG), Rockville, MD, USA
e-mail: shashi.h.ranganath@kp.org

© The Author(s), under exclusive license to Springer Nature   151
Switzerland AG 2025
J. Shames et al. (eds.), *A Radiologist's Path*,
https://doi.org/10.1007/978-3-031-86882-5_30

knowing a practice's approach to quality assurance and peer learning is paramount. Being a part of a high-quality and well-run practice where standards are maintained and learning is encouraged is essential. Consider asking the practice if there is a peer learning program where radiologists may congregate as a group to learn from others' learning opportunities and how major misses are addressed. Regularly scheduled educational conferences and opportunities for support are essential.

Ease of communication, not only amongst radiologists but between radiologists and referring providers and technologists, may be highly variable in a practice. We all know that being unable to convey an urgent result can be extremely frustrating and time-consuming. Consider asking what communication methods and work-flows, and processes are in place. Is there a HIPAA (Health Insurance Portability and Accountability) compliant text or secure messaging system to relay findings to referring providers? Is there an embedded PACS instant messaging system to share cases with colleagues and check urgent issues from technologists? Do reading room assistants help field phone calls and contact referring physicians to expedite convey-ing results? Is there a chat system through the electronic medical record? Any or all of these can help ease daily workflow and improve patient care by expediting and facilitating inter-provider communication.

Finally, particularly during and post-pandemic, the wellness of physicians in a practice is of the utmost importance. A practice with a robust wellness program, whether it is something as simple as occasional lunches or happy hours so that people can see each other outside of work or larger gatherings like picnics or galas, help facilitate a sense of camaraderie and collegiality. Burnout is on the rise, so feeling close to your colleagues can make all the difference personally and professionally.

Part III
After Starting Your First Job

Chapter 31
Preparing for Your First Day on the Job

Shashi Ranganath, Wilbur Chang, and Ainsley MacLean

Preparing for your First Day on the Job

As you envision your first day in your new job, think optimistic, positive, and confident thoughts. It will be a remarkable career in an engaging and rewarding specialty you have worked extremely hard for. Congratulations! Having said all that, we often tell our new radiologists that the first few months in a new job, whether it is your first or a transition mid-career, can feel like running through water. This is primarily due to having new technical systems to navigate and new referring providers, colleagues, and technologists' names to learn, all in the context of busy clinical coverage. So go easy on yourself and expect your first few weeks to have slightly longer days than you will for the remainder of your career.

If you can moonlight during your fellowship, we recommend that, as the more cases, clinical scenarios, and pathology are seen, the better. This allows you to sign final reports, use different dictation or PACS (picture archiving and communication system) systems, and keep up with radiology skills that will help you join any practice. Also, it is always a clever idea to brush up on any skills you may not have recently, for instance, reminding yourself how to do a breast biopsy or fluoroscopic study. Stay current on journals and other educational materials or attend any CME (continuing medical education). Before joining, ask your practice manager if there are any special skills they would like you to brush up on during fellowship.

When you arrive on your first day, give yourself an extra 15 min to show up earlier to account for parking and ID badge challenges so you do not feel flustered. Talk to as many of your future colleagues as possible and ask about a mentorship program to ensure your transition as quickly as possible. When there are departmental events, try to attend these since investing in collegial relationships increases job

S. Ranganath (✉) · W. Chang · A. MacLean
Department of Diagnostic and Interventional Radiology, Mid-Atlantic Permanente Medical Group (MAPMG), Rockville, MD, USA

© The Author(s), under exclusive license to Springer Nature
Switzerland AG 2025
J. Shames et al. (eds.), *A Radiologist's Path*,
https://doi.org/10.1007/978-3-031-86882-5_31

satisfaction. In today's environment, where so many radiology jobs may be virtual, it is essential to maintain as much connection as possible with your practice to ensure you feel satisfied and engaged.

Handling Your First Case as an Attending

Your first case is always a bit nerve-wracking, especially if it is your first chance to sign a report finally. It is important to remember that you will experience tremendous growth during your career so that your words will become increasingly concise and relevant. Also, you must go on to the next case because patients need your care and providers are waiting on their reports. Developing a cadre of colleagues in your group to bounce issues off is essential. It is common for radiologists to show each other cases despite being years out of training, so know that you are not working in a silo.

Chapter 32
Understanding Your Work Environment and System's Information Technology

Shashi Ranganath, Wilbur Chang, and Ainsley MacLean

Understanding Your Work Environment

We recommend jumping right into reading cases as soon as you feel comfortable and get permission, as, ultimately, this is the best way to familiarize yourself with your new practice. Review any materials about standardized reporting, communication, and critical results carefully so that when you encounter them, you are prepared. Remain confident even as things may not always go as expected, and remember that you have spent a long time preparing for this moment.

Be flexible and accommodating with the schedulers and technologists, and do your best to be known as a team player within your group from the get-go. If there are open shifts, offer to cover; if a colleague needs a trade, hop right in. Many impressions are made early on, so if you are viewed as someone who steps up to the plate for a challenge or to cover a colleague, this will remain with you during your career.

If your practice has access to STATdx or other reference materials, ask how to access them. Remember as you hone your reports, always seek to be concise and to the point, without overcalling minor abnormalities of little concern. No one wants to read a long novella, and you want to be known by referring providers as practical and helpful in their practices. Stay up to date on evidence-based care.

As you communicate with your practice leaders, let them know if you have any special skills you would like the group to benefit from or new skills you would like to acquire. For example, if you have a neuroradiology background but know how to read screening mammograms, offer to help. If you have experience or interest in leadership, let that be known early on. The more radiologists take on leadership

S. Ranganath (✉) · W. Chang · A. MacLean
Department of Diagnostic and Interventional Radiology, Mid-Atlantic Permanente Medical Group (MAPMG), Rockville, MD, USA

© The Author(s), under exclusive license to Springer Nature   157
Switzerland AG 2025
J. Shames et al. (eds.), *A Radiologist's Path*,
https://doi.org/10.1007/978-3-031-86882-5_32

roles outside of radiologists, the larger the visibility and the sounding board become for our profession.

Contribute to professional societies as much as possible early on. This will allow you to keep up connections in the community and give you a much bigger picture view of the practice environment outside of your practice. Often, it can be easy only to see the strengths and weaknesses of your practice if you lose sight of what is going on outside.

Understanding Your Systems: EMR, PACS, and Dictation System

The electronic medical record (EMR) plays an increasingly crucial role in the function of radiologists. Previously medical records, being handwritten documents physically stored in a location, were not available for review when interpreting imaging studies. The only information available to the radiologist was written on the imaging prescription. The utilization of electronic medical records, connectivity, and portability of information have made referencing this data more practical. For those fortunate to be interpreting studies within one hospital/organization/integrated healthcare system, data in the EMR can help inform more directed and relevant reports. In such a scenario, the better you know the EMR, the more quickly and efficiently the information you seek can be obtained – like finding a book in a library you know well.

The picture archiving and communication system (PACS) has evolved from physical jackets of film and lightboxes to vast databases of image-related storage and electronic methods of retrieval and display. There are many options for PACS, and all perform similar roles with variations in the number and types of add-on options. From a practical standpoint, the better you understand how to use the system and to use any customizations that decrease the number of actions/clicks, the better off you are. Given the volume of studies typically interpreted in a day, small efficiencies per study will add up over time. Additionally, knowing how to navigate the PACS smoothly will decrease the subconscious distraction of focus from the primary goal of image interpretation caused by performing tasks in the PACS. Take the time upfront to understand the potential shortcuts in using the PACS and stay alert to those tricks you may stumble across during day-to-day use; it is worth it.

Dictation systems are the third key component of the radiologist workflow, which interprets images into a report format. These systems have also moved to digital, partially automated systems. In the quest for improved efficiency and rapid reporting, computer systems and assistive algorithms now commonly perform voice recognition and report generation in real time. Waiting for transcription to return a document after initially sending voice recordings needs to be updated. Moreover, with special devices for voice recognition, opportunities to use multiple functional buttons with both hands and even all extremities with foot pedals are a reality.

As technologies evolve, the trend is to increasingly integrate these systems, EMR/PACS/dictation and, most recently, artificial intelligence. Opening images in PACS is connected to opening the relevant medical record in the EMR and vice versa. The report may contain critical visual information from the PACS and dictated descriptive text. The bottom line is that understanding these systems well will significantly benefit you, the radiologist.

Chapter 33
Handling Your First Case as an Attending

Suzanne McElligott

Regardless of whether you are reading a diagnostic mammogram, signing a body CT scan, or performing a transjugular intrahepatic portosystemic shunt (TIPS), your first case as a new radiology attending will be memorable. This holds if you are starting as an attending physician where you completed your training or starting your first attending job at a new institution. In many ways, it will be very different from what you have encountered before. In other ways, it will be similar. After all, you have been training in radiology for years.

No matter how far out we are from our first case as attendings, we all remember that first day. We experienced a combination of excitement for finally reaching that point in our careers, anxiety about starting a new job and all that entails, and, as physicians, fear that we would make a mistake that could harm a patient.

From my own experience and from what is written by others, there are several ways to approach your first day and your first year with a good combination of excitement and a bit of fear. First, trust in yourself and the training you received [1]. Radiology residency and fellowship training programs are comprehensive and rigorous. They have well-established guidelines for training successful physicians who are competent and ready to practice. By graduating, you have earned your position. You have encountered, through direct experience, reading, and lectures, many situations you will encounter in practice over your career.

A little bit of fear is healthy. It will keep you from being complacent. It and your desire to always be better for your patients will drive you to keep learning and growing as a doctor. And nowadays, you have more tools at your quick disposal than ever to help you develop and grow as an attending. I have known radiology colleagues who utilize STATdx. Internet search engines are available on every computer. And

S. McElligott (✉)
Department of Radiology, Zucker School of Medicine at Hofstra Northwell Health,
Lake Success, NY, USA
e-mail: smcellig@northwell.edu

J. Shames et al. (eds.), *A Radiologist's Path*,
https://doi.org/10.1007/978-3-031-86882-5_33

in combination with your institutional and personal society memberships, you have access to numerous journals with many images to guide you and supplement your hard-earned fund of knowledge.

For management decisions, utilize the appropriate ACR white papers, ACR Appropriateness Criteria, and available atlases for your particular subspecialty. And, of course, use your network of friends and colleagues to discuss a complex case! Have their contact information readily available should you need it. Even a quick phone consult with your former co-fellow or attending can give you the peace of mind you need about a case. We attendings, have all gotten those calls, and are happy to help.

From day one, get to know your colleagues in your and other subspecialties. Learn how to quickly reach them at your institution, whether by phone or through a chat or messaging feature on the PACS. These "view box" consults will be invaluable throughout your career.

Ensure you get to know your support staff as soon as possible, including the IT group, the nurses, technologists, department secretaries, navigators, and front desk staff. They will be an essential resource to help you acclimate and function effectively in your new job. A good working relationship with all these staff members will make your job much more enjoyable. From a personal perspective, one of the most fulfilling aspects of my job is knowing that I am working as a team with a large group of colleagues to provide the best care possible for my patients.

On your first day, expect to work late. Nearly every radiologist I have asked said they reviewed their first case at least twice before signing it. Several new attendings tell me that they reviewed every case a second time before they signed off anything during that first week. This undoubtedly kept them at work much later than they would have preferred, and it is probably not sustainable for the long term. But it gave them much-needed peace of mind for those first few days. Even if you don't plan to review every case again before signing off, anticipate the long workday. There are many inefficiencies built into learning new systems and processes. Try to get a good night of sleep before your first day and plan accordingly for food and childcare needs, among other necessities. You do not want to feel more rushed than necessary on that first day.

Be patient with yourself [2]. The first day and many days during that first year can be daunting and overwhelming. But it does get easier—know that. First, allow yourself extra time to review a case whenever possible. Allow yourself to get a second opinion consult. Allow yourself to acknowledge, even to the patient, that you do not know the answer but will find out for them. In medicine, we are learning every day. It's just that the learning curve is steeper as you start as a new attending. When you encounter cases or pathologies, you have not seen before, read about them and feel you will know the answers the next time you meet them.

There is only one first case and one first day as an attending, but throughout your career, there will be many first times that you encounter a particular issue or situation. Utilizing the tools you set in place on day, one will allow you to face these challenges as they arise and will set you (and your patients) up for success over the course of your career.

References

1. Thomas B. Lessons learned during my first year as an attending physician. ACEP Now. November 24, 2019. https://www.acepnow.com/article/lessons-learned-during-my-first-year-as-an-attending-physician/2/?singlepage=1
2. Babatunde F. What i have learned in my first year as an attending. Doximity Op-Med. December 5, 2018. https://opmed.doximity.com/articles/what-i-have-learned-in-my-first-year-as-an-attending

Chapter 34
When to Ask for Help?

Suzanne McElligott

It has become much easier to obtain a second opinion or seek assistance on a case in radiology. Many practices now have a picture archiving and communication system (PACS) chat or messaging features that allow radiologists to consult online colleagues immediately. In large practice groups, several subspecialized colleagues are usually available to help you with a case. Nevertheless, to some degree, the mental-emotional hurdle to ask for help persists for many of us.

Asking for help at work takes work. That holds for every practice stage—as a medical student, resident, new attending, and seasoned senior attending. But new attendings may need help to request assistance. New attendings are no longer "in training." They have reached the hard-earned stage when they are expected to know the answers. The buck now stops with them.

New attendings are pressured to prove themselves worthy of their position. Sometimes that pressure is self-imposed (and includes imposter syndrome when physicians feel self-doubt or fear of being perceived as less intelligent or less competent than their peers) [1, 2]. This has been found to occur at the start of new jobs [1]. Sometimes, the pressure is external in the group's culture or in the practice's logistics. No one wants to be the one trying to reach their colleague (who is not on call) in the middle of the night with questions about a case.

This situation is uncomfortable for new and experienced attendings alike. One main difference between new attendings and more experienced attendings, however, is that the latter has seen a larger volume of cases over the course of their career, which makes it easier to feel confident that a patient falls into a challenging or unique category and therefore is more worthy of the SOS call.

S. McElligott (✉)
Department of Radiology, Zucker School of Medicine at Hofstra Northwell Health, Lake Success, NY, USA
e-mail: smcellig@northwell.edu

J. Shames et al. (eds.), *A Radiologist's Path*,
https://doi.org/10.1007/978-3-031-86882-5_34

New and senior attendings will likely know when a case is acute enough to ask for a second opinion. Our radiology training is well designed to teach us to recognize those cases. New attendings, however, may feel they should be able to handle the acute case independently precisely because the findings and management of such cases were well ingrained throughout training.

For new attendings trying to decide when to call for help, my advice goes back to the original guiding principle in medicine, "primum non nocere" (Hippocrates), first, do no harm [3]. As physicians, we all took the Hippocratic Oath. The weight of these words never diminishes. When you encounter a case where you need assistance to ensure your patient will receive the correct diagnosis or treatment, you should ask for help, period. No matter what repercussions might ensue, you must do the right thing for the patient.

It would be best if you took your time to read and learn more about all of these cases to supplement your knowledge base. Make it your goal to be the person the next new attending in your group will call for help with a similar issue. And know that even your senior radiology colleagues will need your help with a case at one point or another.

References

1. Chen C. Doctor, who? Reflecting on impostor syndrome in medical learners. Can Fam Physician. 2020 Oct;66(10):e268–9.
2. Clance PR, Imes SA. The imposter phenomenon in high achieving women: dynamics and therapeutic intervention. Psychother Theory Res Pract. 1978;15(3):241.
3. Hippocrates. Oath of Hippocrates. In: Miles S, editor. In The Hippocratic Oath and the ethics of medicine. New York: Oxford University Press; 2004. p. xiii–xiv.

Chapter 35
Billing and Insurances, RVUs, and Other Revenue Streams

Pranav Suri and Lauren C. Pringle

Billing/Insurance

Radiology billing is a team-based approach that requires cooperation from radiologists, medical coders, technologists, and sometimes ordering providers. While this may seem tedious at times, this critical part of the radiologist's workday is vital for accuracy, appropriate reimbursement, and compliance with laws and regulations. Not only does proper coding ensure that radiologists and their practices are reimbursed, but it also helps us make sure that we are truthful and not committing any healthcare fraud.

Radiology billing largely depends on good documentation of the patient's history and the type of service provided. Medical coders translate the indication and type of study documented in the radiologist's report into diagnosis and procedural codes. Billing is based on matching the International Classification of Diseases (ICD) ("diagnosis code") and Current Procedural Terminology (CPT) codes ("procedure" or "service code"). ICD codes identify *why* service was performed, and CPT codes determine *what* service was performed. Mismatched ICD and CPT codes usually cause claim denials, and thinking about how dictations translate into codes is essential for appropriate billing.

ICD codes are used to justify a medical service by identifying diagnoses, health conditions or problems, abnormal findings, signs and symptoms, and injuries. Radiologists are not expected to assign a diagnosis code to patient history or study. Occasionally, study requests will come with the ICD code alone as the survey indicates, and those that perform procedures may need to select diagnoses and codes

P. Suri
University of Missouri – Columbia School of Medicine, Columbia, MO, USA

L. C. Pringle (✉)
Department of Radiology, University of Missouri – Columbia, Columbia, MO, USA
e-mail: laurenpringle@health.missouri.edu

when submitting surgical pathology requests and other orders, so basic familiarity with the system is helpful. Principles of the ICD-10 system currently in use in the United States consist of 3–7 characters: the first three characters identify the category; the fourth through sixth characters identify descriptors such as location, severity, and cause; and the last character is an extension, such as "encounter after treatment" or "sequela." The ICD system is maintained by the World Health Organization (WHO), and the tenth version has nearly 70,000 different codes.

CPT codes indicate which service was performed, and the system is maintained and updated by the American Medical Association (AMA). Each radiologic study is translated into a five-digit CPT code, which calculates physician payment. CPT codes also vary based on details; for instance, a CT abdomen and pelvis without contrast *(74176)* is coded differently from a CT abdomen and pelvis with contrast *(74177)*, and both are coded differently from a CT abdomen and pelvis pre- and post-contrast *(74178)*. Thus, the radiologist needs to include all details about the type of study performed. For radiographs, the most crucial element for coding is a number of distinct views (lateral, AP, etc.), not merely the number of images because sometimes multiple images are taken per individual view. For MRI/CT, whether the acquisitions were non-contrast, pre–/post-contrast, or just with contrast is most important. Including a specific checklist of organs or structures for each exam type is crucial for an ultrasound. For procedures, detailed descriptions of the steps taken can help coders accurately capture the case's complexity. For example, the number of passes within a vessel and the number of vessels cannulated are details that may change the CPT codes and modifiers and thus reimbursement and billing of the case. For all types of cases, structured report templates are one way to ensure that all details required for coding/billing are included and are increasingly utilized by practices and radiologists.

When CPT codes are priced, they are divided into professional and technical fees. The professional fee reflects the work of the interpreting radiologist and includes the report, interpretation, and time. The technical price consists of the equipment, supplies, and personnel necessary to obtain the study. Radiologist income is often highly based on professional fee revenue, and the technical fee revenue goes to the imaging facility/equipment owner. Many private practice groups still own their imaging equipment, and the partner radiologists then receive a portion of the technical fee after paying their share of the cost ("buy-in"). However, hospitals or other groups increasingly may have partial or complete ownership of the equipment and will earn income from the technical fee as a result.

As aforementioned, whether payers accept charges for radiologic services depends on properly matched ICD-10 and CPT codes. For example, it follows that a patient with right lower quadrant abdominal pain *(ICD, R10.31)* and fever would get a CT abdomen and pelvis with contrast *(CPT, 74177)*. Appropriate coding of the patient presentation and service requested depends on the clinical history documentation. If the clinical history for the same patient were instead "rule out appendicitis," Medicare may deny the claim because the record does not capture medical necessity. This is because study indications listing uncertain diagnoses only (such as "rule out" or "concern for") are problematic if the study ends up being negative for that diagnosis. If the study is found to be positive for appendicitis, then the diagnosis code for appendicitis would apply and match with the CPT code for the CT. However, if the CT is negative for appendicitis or other acute pathologies, this study may be denied due to the absence of concrete signs/symptoms that are codable. In such circumstances, the radiology team must obtain a further history from the patient or electronic medical record. Additional history (signs and symptoms) can be obtained by the radiologist or technologist from the medical chart, patient, or ordering provider and included in the report to aid in filing the claim. Some coders may have access to the clinical chart and may be able to obtain the necessary clinical information, but this varies by practice and is usually less efficient. In this example, if the CT technologist spoke with the patient and found out they had right lower quadrant pain and fever for 24 h, this would be appropriate and helpful information to include in the report. On the other hand, if the radiologist just made an educated guess that the patient had these symptoms and included that in the report without verifying with the patient, ordering provider, or chart, this would be considered billing fraud and could have significant consequences for the practice and radiologist. Many practices thus have technologists ask the patient about their symptoms, duration, and any other basic info when the service is rendered.

Most studies are paid for by Medicare/Medicaid or through insurance companies. Patients may also pay cash ("self-pay") or be eligible for charity care through the facility/institution, although this is less common. The practice or institution sets charges. These usually found on a "chargemaster" document. While charges are generally the same for all patients regardless of the payer, different insurance companies have different contracted payment rates for specific services based on negotiations between the payer and facility. Medicare/Medicaid rates are specified by the Medicare Physician Fee Schedule (MPFS). Self-pay patients are often able to negotiate a cash discount with the facility. Many specific charges and rates vary by year and continue to evolve, such as with new rules related to price transparency (2019) and the No Surprises Act (2022). However, all insurance companies and Medicare/Medicaid use ICD/CPT codes to determine coverage for a service, which will likely remain consistent for some time.

Preauthorization is a step in the billing process that is becoming increasingly common, especially in outpatient radiology. For more and more cross-sectional exams and procedures, preapproval is required by a patient's insurance company before performing a test, exam, or procedure to ensure insurance coverage. This can cause a delay between ordering and scheduling a study and may limit same-day add-on exams such as MRIs and procedures. Insurance companies will verify medical necessity by matching ICD and CPT codes before the exam, rather than after the fact. Usually, this process is managed by referring providers and scheduling/ancillary staff rather than radiologists or patients themselves.

RVUs/Reimbursement

The United States primarily operates on a fee-for-service model for healthcare reimbursement. Attending/private practice physicians are ultimately paid through the MPFS, a pool of money reserved for physician payment, and private insurance. Fee-for-service in radiology translates to payment on a case-volume basis; i.e., the more you read, the more you are paid. Trainees are paid a set salary unrelated to their caseload. Payer approval of properly matched ICD and CPT codes results in reimbursement by translating the CPT code into relative value units (RVUs). RVUs are the basis of physician/practice payment through the resource-based relative value scale (RBRVS), a scale used by the Centers for Medicare and Medicaid Services (CMS) and private insurance. RVUs quantify the relative work, cost, and value of medical services. Nearly every service described by CPT is given a total RVU (RVU_T) according to the following formula [4]:

$$RVU_T = wRVU + RVU_{PE} + RVU_{ME}$$

wRVU is the RVU of physician work ("work RVU"), RVU_{PE} is the RVU of practice expense, and RVU_{ME} is the RVU of malpractice. Medicare payment per RVU can be calculated by multiplying the total RVU by a geographical practice cost index (GPCI) and a conversion factor (CF) that incorporates business adjustment factors and legislation [5].

In addition to being a component of physician reimbursement, the wRVU is a well-described and discussed metric of physician productivity [1, 2]. Each CPT code for radiology exams is assigned a wRVU value that has been adjusted over time. The role of wRVUs in individual radiologist salary varies by type of practice (academic, private practice, hybrid, VA, etc.) and individual approach. The number of wRVUs per study is loosely tied to the complexity of the study. It has been negotiated by the leadership in radiology societies such as the ACR, but over time some studies/procedures have been weighted differently than others. Even so, some of the studies' wRVUs differ from the average time needed to interpret them relative to other studies. For example, the time and effort to solve a complex radiograph compared to a normal MRI will not be reflected in the standard wRVUs assigned to the study. An MRI is generally considered more difficult/complex to interpret compared to radiographs, which is reflected in the assigned wRVU. Furthermore, when a study's wRVU value is adjusted by the RBVRS committee, it is typically "devalued" instead of being assigned a greater value. Thus, the wRVU system is felt by most to not fully capture the effort of an individual radiologist, so many practices have devised ways to equalize the productivity expectations (such as weighting wRVUs by subspecialty), by using other metrics, or a common worklist to avoid emphasizing wRVUs at all.

Increasingly, healthcare payers are looking to reimburse physicians based on quality metrics. Most recently, the Medicare Access and CHIP Reauthorization Act (MACRA) replaced the old Sustainable Growth Rate model with the Quality

Payment Program (QPP). Under QPP, physicians participate in Merit-Based Incentive Payment Systems (MIPS) or Advanced Alternative Payment Models (APMs) to avoid wRVU devaluing. MIPS has four performance categories: quality, promoting interoperability, improvement activities, and cost. Performance in each category is summarized in a single performance score, evaluated on a two-year cycle. Performance scores above a certain threshold may lead to upward payment adjustments. Studies on MIPS have already found that radiologists score higher when using group reporting versus individual reporting, but those that used APMs scored the highest [3]. As a relatively new system, implementation strategies and financial impact are still evolving. They will likely play a more significant role in daily radiologist practice and income in the coming years.

Other Income Streams

Besides reading cases and performing image-guided procedures, radiologists can earn income from specialized training through other avenues. Some radiologists (usually interventional radiologists, neuroradiologists, and musculoskeletal radiologists) will see patients in the clinic before and after their procedures and will bill for those services. Radiologists can consult for companies and earn income and royalties by advising on device research and development. Some radiologists may earn speaking fees as invited lecturers or may be asked to review cases for research or other purposes for an hourly rate. Another common area for side income is to serve as an expert witness in malpractice or criminal cases, where radiologists' expertise can be billed for case review, depositions, or trial testimony. Finally, there is a multitude of "side gigs" for physicians and radiologists outside the more common areas listed above that can contribute to physician income during or after a traditional career in radiology that are beyond the scope of this chapter and range from blogging to real estate investing, among countless other endeavors.

References

1. Duszak R, Muroff LR. Measuring and managing radiologist productivity, part 2: beyond the clinical numbers. J Am Coll Radiol. 2010a;7(7):482–9. https://doi.org/10.1016/j.jacr.2010.01.025.
2. Duszak R, Muroff LR. Measuring and managing radiologist productivity, part 1: clinical metrics and benchmarks. J Am Coll Radiol. 2010b;7(6):452–8. https://doi.org/10.1016/j.jacr.2010.01.026.
3. Rosenkrantz AB, Duszak R, Golding LP, Nicola GN. The alternative payment model pathway to radiologists' success in the merit-based incentive payment system. J Am Coll Radiol. 2020;17(4):525–33. https://doi.org/10.1016/j.jacr.2019.09.016.
4. Smith S. Medicare RBRVS 2009: the physicians' guide. American Medical Association; 2009.
5. Woody IO. The fundamentals of the US Medicare physician reimbursement process. J Am Coll Radiol. 2005;2(2):139–50. https://doi.org/10.1016/j.jacr.2004.07.023.

Chapter 36
The Doctor's Doctor: Working with Colleagues in Other Specialties

Christopher Roth

Often called the "doctor's doctor," radiologists are consultants to other physicians, interpreting complex medical imaging studies and providing diagnoses based on those images (although the CARES Act has increased patient access) [1]. Radiologists act as specialists that other physicians rely on to interpret the findings of a patient's scan accurately. They have extensive training in reading various imaging modalities, allowing them to identify subtle details that might be missed by other doctors. Radiologists can further specialize in specific areas of radiology, providing even deeper expertise in certain body systems. As a consultant, radiologists confer with referring physicians to diagnose the patient's condition. They are key members of the patient's medical care team, often working "behind the scenes." In this sense, the radiologist aids the referring doctor by providing guidance on how the referring doctor does for the patient. Although patients often may never meet the radiologist interpreting their exams, there are areas where patients may have close contact with radiologists. This includes areas like breast imaging and interventional radiology, where radiologists have significant patient contact. It is here where the doctor's doctor becomes the patient's doctor as well.

Generally, referring physicians are looking for clarity, confirmation, or exclusion of a provisional diagnosis and/or compliance with evidence- or consensus-based guidelines. Having said that, the degree to which radiologist consultations serve this clarifying role depends on the way radiologist consultations or reports are phrased or delivered. Examples might help explain how radiologists serve as the doctor's doctor. Consider this scenario in which a patient with an abdominal aortic aneurysm originally 5.7 × 5.6 cm presents to the hospital a month later with an 8.4 × 6.6 cm aneurysm and multiple findings indicating impending rupture that go underappreciated by the non-radiologists (Fig. 36.1). This patient was sick with an infection and

C. Roth (✉)
Jefferson Health & Thomas Jefferson University, Philadelphia, PA, USA
e-mail: Christopher.Roth@jefferson.edu

J. Shames et al. (eds.), *A Radiologist's Path*,
https://doi.org/10.1007/978-3-031-86882-5_36

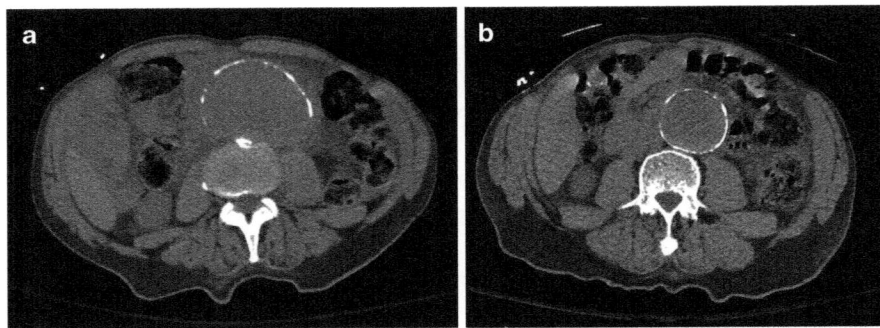

Fig. 36.1 Impending aortic rupture
The first CT image (**a**) through the mid-abdomen performed without contrast shows a very large abdominal aortic aneurysm with a saccular configuration, periaortic haziness, and discontinuous calcifications (arrows) which were not discontinuous on the image from the CT scan 6 weeks earlier (**b**)

had numerous complaints and comorbidities that confused the clinical picture, and the inpatient CT was ordered to identify a source of infection which sounds reasonable under the admitting diagnosis of "sepsis." Numerous radiographic signs portended impending rupture including the hyperdense crescent sign, disruption of mural calcifications, and the development of a saccular configuration, in addition to the abrupt caliber change (Fig. 36.1). However, the significance of these findings was lost on the clinical team, who noted an "increase in size of the aortic aneurysm" with no plan or statement of its clinical significance. A secure message sent to all clinical stakeholders prompted the initial response asking whether a contrast-enhanced study would help which underscored the fact that they missed the point that imaging findings indicated imminent death without any further clarification. However, one resident took this to heart and called the patient's daughter to communicate the dire nature of the patient's situation, and she responded that it "sounds like he's between a rock and a hard place." Two hours later, a code blue was called and the patient expired.

The point is that radiologists need to effectively communicate imaging findings to clinicians without a deep appreciation of imaging findings to convey the deeper meaning that eludes them. Sometimes, this means simply making a diagnosis such as appendicitis on a CT scan to confirm a relatively straightforward diagnosis, and sometimes, it means a more nuanced communication as described above. While clinicians have varying facility with imaging data depending on their respective specialties, operating from the assumption that they have no interpretation skills, the radiologist's role starts with delineating the findings. These findings should be framed in the clinical context with which the clinician is generally familiar and often what prompted them to order the imaging study in the first place. This might include referencing tumor markers such as alpha-fetoprotein or CA 125 in the contexts of chronic liver disease and suspected hepatocellular carcinoma (HCC) and ovarian carcinoma, respectively, or symptoms such as right lower quadrant pain in suspected appendicitis, for example. In other words, the process most effectively starts with enumerating the observations—the clinical observations in the "History" or "Indication" fields of the radiology report and imaging findings in the "Findings" field of the radiology report—as the first step in an exercise in inductive reasoning to arrive at a clinical diagnosis (Fig. 36.2). The next step involves pattern recognition and the ability to craft imaging finding descriptions that fit into established patterns. For example, the description of a "hyperenhancing mass with washout and a capsule appearance in a nodular liver" is diagnostic of an HCC. The hyperenhancing-washout-capsule pattern is typical of an HCC, and, in the setting of a nodular liver (indicating cirrhosis), it is considered diagnostic of HCC. While this might seem straightforward, precision in descriptors is important – simply stating the mass enhances instead of "hyperenhancing" would not provide the specificity to arrive at the diagnosis.

In most cases, the inductive process is not so simple, and generating a differential diagnosis is necessary (from which a favored diagnosis can be highlighted). For example, an occasionally encountered radiologic pattern is "multiple cystic liver lesions" which implicates numerous diagnostic possibilities. In order to manage the numerous diagnostic considerations, a broad approach starting with disease categories helps manage the infinite possibilities. In this example, disease categories would include neoplastic with subcategories including primary and secondary neoplasms, inflammatory, congenital, and traumatic (Fig. 36.3). Of course, the description of the observations is critical to prioritizing among the categories and specific diagnoses, but it is generally worth considering the full breadth of the options, especially with less clinical certainty. For example, emphasizing the "marked" nature of enhancement and fat stranding adjacent to a segment of bowel wall thickening implies an inflammatory etiology. Remember, the audience or reader can and will appreciate the logical stream from observations to disease category aligned with pattern recognition leading to an inductive conclusion. The better the description of the observations or findings corresponds to a pattern, the more likely a diagnostic conclusion will be attainable.

Radiologists also have significant roles in multidisciplinary tumor boards, helping to guide the team on the patient's imaging findings and what role the imaging could have on the patient's staging and treatment. For example, breast radiologists work closely with surgery and oncology services to provide needed information and answer questions that will determine care management plans. Preparing tumor board cases, although time-consuming, also allows the radiologist to review cases she may not have otherwise reviewed, adding to her knowledge base.

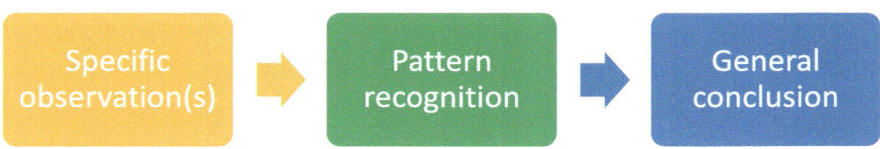

Fig. 36.2 The inductive reasoning process

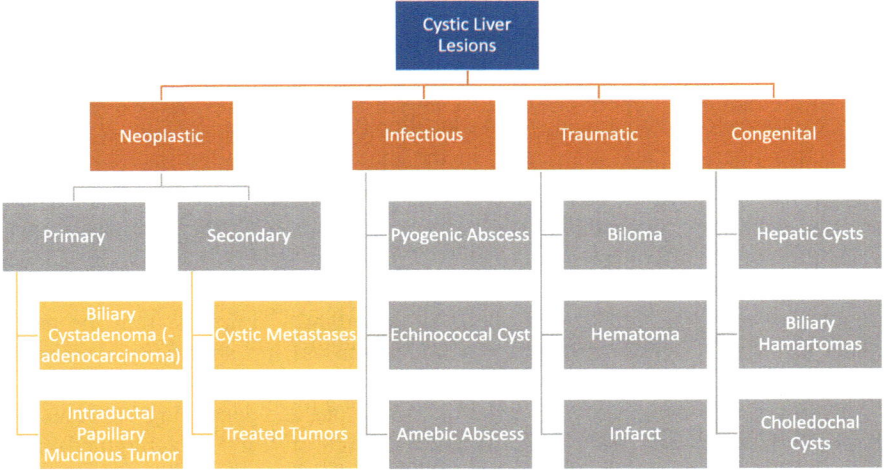

Fig. 36.3 Cystic liver lesion disease category example

A final way radiologists serve as the doctor's doctor is in the role of gatekeeper over medical imaging, helping referring providers from a risk-benefit standpoint in the form of a clinical decision-support role. Radiologists are the experts of medical imaging and which tests would be most beneficial or useful to answer a particular question. It is the radiologist's job to serve as an educator to referring physicians regarding what the most appropriate test might be to arrive at a diagnosis.

It is important for the radiologist to remember that in addition to reading and interpreting the studies on the ever-growing list of exams performed on a given day and meeting turnaround time expectations and RVU goals, he or she *is*, in fact, the doctor's doctor. And with that responsibility comes phone calls or visits to the reading room, outside consultations, and joint care team meetings. Yes, it can be overwhelming, time-consuming, and somewhat intrusive at times, but it is important to remember the privilege of being able to take care of patients and be a part of the medical team, as well as form meaningful relationships with referring colleagues. It's just another reason why radiology is a great choice of specialty.

Reference

1. Mezrich JL, et al. Patient electronic access to final radiology reports: what is the current standard of practice, and is an embargo period appropriate? Radiology. 2021;300(1):187–9.

Chapter 37
What Do I Want from My Radiologist?

Jason Shames, Lisa Zorn, and Kahyun Yoon-Flannery

Being a diagnostic radiologist is a weird job.

It seems straightforward. You can describe the study interpretation of the job in a sentence or two. When asked at a party by a nonmedical acquaintance what you do, you can say, "I read MRIs, CTs, and ultrasound studies" or something similar. We interpret imaging studies. We write reports. We communicate those findings to doctors (mostly, except in mammography). That's it.

This is how we get paid. Period. Whatever else we may do, we don't get paid by insurance companies or the government (Medicare/Medicaid) for it. We may get paid a small stipend by hospitals or academic institutions for our administrative responsibilities, or we might have grant money for research projects. But the bottom line RVU generator is "film" reading.

Many referring doctors think that's ALL we do. And many administrators feel that this is all that matters. Even some radiologists who run large practices may get seduced into thinking RVUs are all that matters.

The consequences of narrowing the broad flow of radiology service to the pinpoint garden hose spout of film reading create massive pressure on a single point: We can't miss significant findings.

J. Shames (✉)
Department of Radiology, Jefferson Health & Thomas Jefferson University,
Philadelphia, PA, USA
e-mail: jason.shames@jefferson.edu

L. Zorn
Department of Radiology, Jefferson Health & Thomas Jefferson University,
Philadelphia, PA, USA

K. Yoon-Flannery
MD Anderson Cancer Center at Cooper, Cooper Medical School of Rowan University,
Camden, NJ, USA

At some point early in your career, you will miss a finding. You'll miss plenty of results no one cares about, including you. But there will come a time when you will learn of missing an important finding. One that has or could have had enormous consequences for the patient. You will look back at the case and may have no idea why the finding didn't occur to you then. At least, that's been my experience—more than once.

When viewed through this microscope of "all that matters is your report," this experience of missing a case can become extremely painful.

I remember the meme, "You had one job." So ominous.

"You had one job" (!)

This can lead to early burnout.

It gets worse. The more subspecialized you become, based on many extra hours of training, reading, and lectures in your subspecialized field, the more likely you are to read cases for subspecialized expert clinicians who have mastered imaging interpretation in their narrow field of expertise.

For example, a neuroradiology will read many imaging studies for neurologists and neurosurgeons. Imaging is of significant significance to both fields, neurosurgeons especially. They operate on the spine, the spinal cord, and the brain!

Many also do endovascular work using cerebral angiography, which used to be done by neuroradiologists exclusively.

Because they have to have the best possible knowledge of what they will encounter before operating on a brain or spinal cord, what kind of surgeons would they be if they weren't at least somewhat good at interpreting MRIs and CTs on their own? What kind of neurosurgeon doesn't look at the images? What sort of neurosurgeon trusts in whatever the diagnostic radiologist says? Even if the diagnostic radiologist was an internationally renowned academic neuroradiologist?

So, what role does, say, a neuroradiologist play here? At best, you can add a bit of extra knowledge. But rest assured, all the aspects of the imaging that matter to how they will approach the lesion in question are elements they will address before surgery. They will know just how much blood to expect from a lesion, including whether or not preoperative embolization will be helpful. They will analyze the studies to anticipate the extent of venous sinus invasion. They will look for the size of the tumor spread throughout the skull base neural foramina.

You can only fail to do what they do.

"You had one job" (!)

And yet, you can be precious to even the most sophisticated and specialized referring docs by viewing your job through the broad lens of what you do.

One way is to see yourself as an imaging consultant.

As a full-fledged imaging consultant, you take responsibility for helping your fellow doctors to use imaging to answer their clinical questions best. This includes helping them choose the best study for their specific patient with her medical needs at this particular point in her diagnostic workup or treatment. It means ensuring the studies you get are of the highest quality within the limitations of the imaging equipment you work with. It means letting them know of other imaging options, sometimes outside of where you work, to get them what they need.

It means reviewing outside MRIs and CTs and pointing out the advantages and limitations based on the different equipment and protocols used elsewhere. (This is a huge one!) Even the most sophisticated of our referring doctors often have no idea why the outside study they got from an MRI of East Whoknowswhere looks so different from the ones they get from your magnets. They usually don't realize that the lesion not seen in that study did not go away; it just wasn't visible due to different protocols or limitations of another scanner. There's often little to no reimbursement for second opinions on outside studies. Yet, you can massively increase the respect and confidence of your referring docs by helping them understand these, especially the advantages and limitations of the different equipment or imaging protocols used.

A regular presence at tumor boards with significant contributions when imaging questions arise also makes a tremendous impact on the trust and respect with which those doctors who attend will view you. This counts. Your radiation oncology colleagues often could use your expertise even though we still need to get paid for time helping them plan their treatments. If you have the time, I suggest volunteering to assist them. What you can learn from them, in return, will help you better interpret studies on cancer patients treated with various forms of radiation.

Yes, you need to do your best to read studies the best you can. Many publications have addressed how best to do this, including ones on style ("be brief where possible," "answer the clinical question," "use RADS systems whenever applicable, as part of a general strategy of relying on evidence-based medicine for recommendations").

But clinicians want more than that. And when you are reading for specialists who are likely very good amateur radiologists about their narrow field of expertise, your value will be much more as a broad imaging consultant than as a "film reader" alone.

Your interpretative abilities become FAR more critical for the primary care physician and other primary care providers, such as physician assistants and nurse practitioners. ER physicians sit somewhere in between primary care docs and specialists. In these cases, liaison is your second most important job as an imaging consultant. Your reads and guidance are needed to get this patient to a surgeon, or to avoid consulting a surgeon, or to get more labs related to such-and-such conditions, or to focus clinical history on work-related exposure to airborne pathogens like asbestos or silica. Judicious recommendations for additional imaging, using evidence-based guidelines whenever you can, are also crucial here.

Our last bit of advice is "don't leave them hanging." Try not to make observations that might leave them more confused than when you started, and when commenting on findings, be concise with what the finding is and what the next steps should be.

Chapter 38
Creating Good Relationships with Referring Doctors

Jason Shames, Lisa Zorn, and Kahyun Yoon-Flannery

Being a diagnostic radiologist is a fun and weird job.

So how to do this? I'm going to state several obvious factors first.

Be available.

Be courteous.

Be helpful.

Be generous with your time.

Simple, right?

But, but, but. ... .

Job pressures conspire to make you want to avoid following these easy prescriptions but these are what make us the doctor's doctor and the patient's advocate.

The time you carve out to achieve each of these goals will not only make it worthwhile, but it will make the other items on this list more achievable.

Here's our advice.

One, make yourself available. By calling clinicians more frequently than necessary and encouraging them to call you, you are much more likely to have much higher quality, non-strained, and often enjoyable interactions with them. Phone calls with referring docs have often been my highest source of job satisfaction on a given day.

J. Shames (✉)
Department of Radiology, Jefferson Health & Thomas Jefferson University,
Philadelphia, PA, USA
e-mail: jason.shames@jefferson.edu

L. Zorn
Department of Radiology, Jefferson Health & Thomas Jefferson University,
Philadelphia, PA, USA

K. Yoon-Flannery
MD Anderson Cancer Center at Cooper, Cooper Medical School of Rowan University,
Camden, NJ, USA

© The Author(s), under exclusive license to Springer Nature
Switzerland AG 2025
J. Shames et al. (eds.), *A Radiologist's Path*,
https://doi.org/10.1007/978-3-031-86882-5_38

As rewarding as picking up a problematic diagnosis may be, it can be even more satisfying to discuss it with the patient's doctor. That way, they get to know just how expert you are. And they will see you as the stand-up, responsible, decent human you are. Once you've earned that respect, your interactions with them will become far more enjoyable. Knowing several of your referring docs well can improve your job satisfaction.

Be courteous. We are all facing tremendous stressors, and being courteous and professional to key to building strong working relationships and gaining the confidence from our referring providers and their team members, patients, and our own team members.

Be helpful. Taking the time to help a doctor with a confusing report or a second opinion has always been time well spent. I get an opportunity to quickly get a clinical history that may have been difficult to extract from the electronic medical record. I learn the role imaging plays in helping them treat this patient. I become a better doctor.

What if the referring doctor calls to complain about a missed diagnosis? Okay, these calls are unpleasant at best. Sometimes, the referring docs are angry, and the communication is borderline abusive.

Let's say this is **not the preferred way to learn**. But you must learn. Sometimes, you know how to focus more on condition "X" because it's more important to them than you had previously surmised. Sometimes, you realize that your focus on condition Y, as vital as you thought it was, was unimportant to them.

But you learn. Stay humble and allow the experience to make you better. Know you are doing your best and we all make mistakes.

Be generous with your time.

This is a tricky one. I suggest working on your time management skills to allow extra time spent communicating with referring docs on challenging cases. Part of this means cutting down time on easy studies. Save your time and energy when it's needed.

I've repeatedly learned that talking with referring docs about challenging cases is helpful. First, I learn a lot from these interactions. Second, I earn respect from them, even in cases where I don't know the answers. I've learned they often don't expect that from me. If they expect a level of expertise I don't have, I let them know I don't and then try to direct them to where they can get it. Sometimes, I'm lucky enough to have colleagues in my practice for whom I need their expert opinion. Other times, I need to refer them to local academic attendings from whom I've learned a bit about this topic but who I know can give them the expert opinion they need.

Angry customers.

Have you worked in retail? Many of you have not. Have you been an IT worker? If you've never received unbridled anger in your work, welcome to radiology.

Anger comes from a combination of reality not meeting expectations (which may be unrealistic) plus a sense on the part of the angry person that they've been rooked, cheated, jerked around, or something similar.

Expectations must be met to result in satisfaction. Expectations regularly not met can result in resignation.

For these to result in anger, however, the person has to feel you wronged them in failing to meet their (again, possibly unrealistic) expectations.

Okay, so how to deal with the angry phone call?

Recognize their anger, and for a few minutes, abandon your side and fully understand theirs. Empathy goes a long way to understanding and overcoming one's anger. Take their anger as a sign that they need your attention. In this case, choose to give it to them, fully. If their anger is coming from a miss or clear fault of your own, show humility and own it. While no one has the right to belittle or degrade you, we all have the opportunity to do the right thing, and being respectful and professional is always in your and the patient's best interest. Don't let someone else's belligerence drag you down to their level. Once the situation is over, it is important to acknowledge how you are feeling in that moment and allow your self to heal and move past it.

Chapter 39
Educating Residents

Theresa Kaufman

As physicians, we are all educators. The word "doctor" comes from the Latin word for *teacher*. This may be by educating patients, medical students, and residents/fellow trainees. Teaching radiology residents is rewarding but can also have its challenges [1, 2]. It requires a unique skill set for imparting a vast amount of knowledge to an adult learner and requires you to stay up to date with research and ever-changing technology. Additionally, taking the time to educate others may come at a cost when balancing productivity expectations and clinical work [1]. In this chapter, we will discuss some factors to consider when deciding between practice settings and tips for getting started when working with residents.

Value Added

No matter the practice setting you join after training, most groups will seek someone who can add value in one way or another. "Value" may come in the form of administrative duties, research/innovation, trainee education, and clinical excellence. When trying to figure out how *you* can add value, the best advice that I can give is to ask yourself: What are my priorities? This will help you to focus your efforts on what is truly important to you. If helping to advance the field by educating our future colleagues is one of your goals, read on.

T. Kaufman (✉)
Department of Radiology, Thomas Jefferson University Hospitals, Philadelphia, PA, USA
e-mail: Theresa.kaufman@jefferson.edu

© The Author(s), under exclusive license to Springer Nature Switzerland AG 2025
J. Shames et al. (eds.), *A Radiologist's Path*,
https://doi.org/10.1007/978-3-031-86882-5_39

Factors to Consider

Practice Setting

Different practice types offer the opportunity to teach residents. Some are larger academic institutions where participating in resident education is a daily expectation. However, these days more and more of those traditional educational institutions also have community-based practices where teaching may look different in quantity and type. There are also hybrid private practices affiliating with residency programs at community-based hospitals. Across the board, clinical volumes over the years have increased, changing demands on workflow versus the education of trainees. Incorporating teaching into a busy clinic can be challenging. Depending on practice type, the expectations of productivity versus daily instruction at the workstation versus didactic lecturing may vary, and it is essential to ask. Knowing the expectations upfront will help you to decide what type of practice setting is best for you and help you to meet your goals.

Recent Changes

Resident education is a constantly evolving target based on trainee needs and learning styles [3]. Moreover, several factors have resulted in broad shifts in how resident education is delivered in daily readouts and conferences over the past decade. Recently, pandemic-related social distancing requirements have led to remote or hybrid readout sessions, altering reading room workflow and the ability for trainees to observe and learn search pattern recognition from faculty. The change from oral board examinations to the multiple-choice CORE and certifying exams has modified the learning emphasis to follow the current testing format rather than focus on description and discussion. We have seen increased learner requests for interactive experiences such as audience response and case-based learning and increased access to web-based prerecorded lectures and modules [4]. This may result in less necessity for traditional didactic PowerPoint lectures from faculty with a shift toward interactive case conferences.

Tips

No matter where you end up, if you are involved in resident teaching, you can significantly impact the quality of their educational experience and, in turn, their future practice. Below are a few tips, some that can be performed on a divisional level for each rotation and others that are more individualized. These tips are not related to the radiology instruction but rather the interaction with residents to help support their learning and transitions through training:

- Be organized and set expectations. Send out the schedule, rotation expectations, resident objectives/responsibilities, etc., before each block. Orient/reorient the residents to the rotation so that they know of any changes and where to find pertinent information. This allows for a good foundation upon which to start each block.
- Remember that each resident will need different types of support, even those at the same PGY/R level. Everyone comes in with varying experiences and abilities—having a "one-size-fits-all" approach to every resident may limit your capacity to help each reach their potential. Try to meet them where they are, and allow for graded levels of responsibility and independence through the rotation and over the years. Let them know they are supported and can come to you with questions.
- If you see a good teaching case, save it while thinking about it. The day gets busy, and you may need to remember to do so later. Solid case collections will help you build conferences and quickly reference good examples for at-the-workstation teaching.
- Feedback.

  - Take the time to let residents know what they are doing well and what can be improved. If needed, do this at the midpoint of the rotation so that they have ample time to incorporate your feedback before the end of the block and then again at the end of every course.
  - Feedback is a two-way street: give residents an avenue to provide constructive criticism for the rotation and discuss what worked well for them. This not only allows them to feel heard and validated but also helps them to improve continuously.

- Beyond teaching didactics and the clinical aspects of reading images, we are role models for residents for professionalism, work ethic, and patient interactions. Set a good example.
- Ask the residents how they are doing. You'll learn a lot about who they are as people.

References

1. Jamadar DA, Carlos R, Caoili EM, Pernicano PG, Jacobson JA, Patel S, Noroozian M, Dong Q, Bailey JE, Patterson SK, Klein KA, Good JD, Kazerooni EA, Reed Dunnick N. Estimating the effects of informal radiology resident teaching on radiologist productivity: what is the cost of teaching? Acad Radiol. 2005;12(1):123–8. https://doi.org/10.1016/j.acra.2004.11.006.
2. Cohen MD, Gunderman RB, Frank MS, Williamson KB. Challenges facing radiology educators. J Am Coll Radiol. 2005;2(8):681–7. https://doi.org/10.1016/j.jacr.2005.03.008.

3. Griffith B, Kadom N, Straus CM. Radiology education in the 21st century: threats and opportunities. J Am Coll Radiol. 2019;16(10):1482–7. ISSN 1546-1440. https://doi.org/10.1016/j.jacr.2019.04.003.
4. Sugi MD, Kennedy TA, Shah V, et al. Bridging the gap: interactive, case-based learning in radiology education. Abdom Radiol. 2021;46:5503–8. https://doi.org/10.1007/s00261-021-03147-z.

Chapter 40
Interactions with Technologists, Support Staff, Nursing, and Administration

Thea Moran and Christopher Roth

You want to be a radiologist and, congratulations, there are plenty of positions available. However, there are other members of the radiology ecosystem, namely, technologists, support staff, nurses, and administrators. It is imperative that each radiology ecosystem member understands the value that each member brings to the department and have empathy for their stressors and potential triggers; this chapter is an applied discussion of communication, professionalism, and systems-based practice in the radiology department, 3 of the 6 Accreditation Council for Graduate Medical Education (ACGME) residency competencies. While it is important to understand each team member's roles and perspectives, at the same time, it has become increasingly difficult to build relationships with your team members because of increased workflow demands, the rise of remote work, and the complexity of staff hiring within organizations. Since both the ACGME and American Board of Radiology (ABR) require graduating residents to demonstrate an understanding of communication, professionalism, and systems-based practice, you may consider this chapter a brief lesson in these competencies as applied to the four aforementioned stakeholders. You're welcome.

T. Moran (✉)
MyriadMD Radiology Consulting, LLC, New Orleans, LA, USA
e-mail: tmoran@myriadmd.com

C. Roth
Jefferson Health & Thomas Jefferson University, Philadelphia, PA, USA
e-mail: Christopher.Roth@jefferson.edu

Technologists

Build a strong relationship with these people because these are the radiology eco-system members you will most frequently interact with. To quote John Chalmers DaCosta: "In order to get the best results, not only must the apparatus be good, but the 'man' who uses it must be expert. Pictures taken by an unskilled man lack clear-ness of outline and may lead to erroneous conclusions" [1]. Radiology technologists (RTs) are experts at getting the best diagnostic images by using their patient care and equipment use training, so radiologists do not come to "erroneous conclusions."

RTs and radiologists have similarities and differences. Both RTs and radiologists have opportunities to get a quality "stamp of approval," by either the ARRT (for RTs) or the ABR (MDs). Both RTs and MDs get separate licenses for each state they want to practice, and both have annual continuing education requirements. Both professions have societies that offer educational opportunities and advocacy in exchange for dues paid. However, RTs are usually hired by hospitals or healthcare systems, while radiologists have traditionally been hired by practices, or depart-ments, that contract with hospitals (with a recent trend toward hiring radiologists as hospital employees or by corporations that contract with hospitals/healthcare orga-nizations). There are, however, two more fundamental differences between RTs and radiologists. The two differences are in their required program competencies and certifying examination content. There are six primary and eight post primary certifi-cates that the ARRT offers, each with their respective pathways [2, 3]. Each path-way has an examination with its own "fair game" content [4]. Diagnostic radiology ACGME competencies [5] and ABR examination content [6] are discussed on their respective websites. Competencies and exam content are clearly different for radi-ologists and RTs.

RTs are like your car: treat them with care and they'll take care of you. Much of this paragraph is also applicable to support staff, nursing, and administration. The biggest thing: control any attitude you may be tempted to have at any given moment. No good comes from being disrespectful to an RT. Never treat an RT in a way that could be interpreted as they are less intelligent than you; we differ in training and the way we add value to the ecosystem, not in intelligence. Next, if they ask a ques-tion, answer it politely. This is the best way to look at it: it is possible that by them asking this question now, they are potentially avoiding a situation down the road that can cause more time and trouble than the time it takes to answer the question now. There may also be times when they don't know something but, remember, they have a fund of knowledge and experience that you do not have and often know things you do not. In a worst-case scenario, treating RTs disrespectfully can cause them to fear asking you anything which can lead to patient care repercussions. These are thoughts on what not to do, but what can you actively do to build your relationships? Whenever I travel, I bring back something (i.e., tasty treats) for the RTs and other staff. This comes in especially handy when there is not much time to talk and build relationships and/or if RTs have felt demeaned by doctors in the past.

Also, I bring microwaveable lunches which provides an excuse to go into the break-room so I can spend time talking with them. When I do these things, I nonverbally communicate that I value them as professionals and human beings (and takes minimal time out of my work schedule).

Support Staff

Medical billers and coders are vital to the financial health of any patient care entity. After a radiology report is generated, the coders translate this information into standardized codes, i.e., ICD-10-CM or Current Procedural Terminology. The medical biller then submits the coded records to the payor (health insurance company, Medicare, etc.) for reimbursement. Both jobs require accuracy, but how accurately they perform their jobs, and the amount and speed of reimbursement, is contingent on your report quality. Money is left on the table if a report omits information that the coders/billers could use in a claim. If the report is unclear, they will call you.

Clerical desk staff perform patient intake duties, such as taking the completed history forms and insurance information. These duties are important for workflow and the organization's financial health. Clerks are an easy group to talk to as you would expect from someone dealing with the public. I don't remember ever having to interact with a clerk about patient care, so I imagine it doesn't happen often for most people. Scheduling may be done by the clerk or by someone dedicated to that duty. Schedulers can also operate remotely from the location they are scheduling for. Scheduling can be a tough job with potential to negatively impact workflow. I have never had to speak to a scheduler because I have not had a problem where I felt I had to. But if a problem was to come up that was ongoing and giving me grief, I would positively go through the chain of command and spin the "complaint" so the listener would hear how the problem negatively impacts the organization's mission and not make it personal.

Nursing

Radiology nurses have two main roles: start IVs and peri−/intraprocedural sedation care. The most common settings where a patient will be needing an IV are in CT or MRI (if they are getting IV contrast) or in IR (and sometimes MRI) where sedation is often needed. Registered nurses are the nurses that you are most likely to see working in radiology. Aspiring registered nursing students obtain either an Associates or Bachelor of Science in Nursing degree from a school approved by the state board to which they are applying. When a nurse is close to graduating, they apply to the board in the state where they want to work; they then take, and pass, the National Council Licensure Exam for Registered Nurses (NCLEX-RN), whereupon they will be placed on the registry of licensed nurses for the jurisdiction of the licensing body (i.e., the state) [7]. This process differs from physicians and technologists in that nurses get their "seal of approval" from their state boards, and we get ours from a national association (i.e., ABR, ARRT) and then apply to the state boards for licensing. Advanced practice registered nurses (AKA nurse practitioners) can be found working in the radiology department, although it is mostly in IR. APRNs need either a Master of Science in Nursing (MSN) or a Doctor of Nursing Practice (DNP) to be awarded an APRN certificate. APRNs must pass an exam in their area of specialization from a certifying organization [8]; there is no radiology certificate in nursing. APRNs are required to obtain continuing education credits, among other requirements, to maintain their state licenses; they must maintain both their RN and APRN licensures while working as an APRN.

Much of what I discussed in the RT section in paragraph 3 is at least doubly true when dealing with radiology nurses. Radiology is unique in that the RN use in the radiology department is minor compared with other departments, and, depending on the practice situation, departments can function without them. Nurses can feel unappreciated in the radiology department which can affect how the radiology ecosystem functions as a team. It is important to recognize the potential for this dynamic and not inadvertently hit a nerve; as I said above, treat them empathetically and have respect for their training and what they add to patient care. If problems are significant and affect the department's mission, hopefully you will have somebody in a managerial position who can help remedy the situation (or at least give it perspective that will make it more tolerable).

Administration

These are the people who oversee either the entire radiology practice/department (practice directors/chairpeople) or portions of it (the main ones are residency program directors, radiology directors, nurse managers). These relationships are, arguably, the second most important to develop (I say second because you will interact with RTs more). Practice directors/chairpeople manage the radiologists (hire/fire, contracts, scheduling, complaints, productivity). Practice directors/chairpeople secure equipment and/or hire additional personnel as the budget allows. Practice directors usually have dedicated management training, if not an MBA; managerial training for chairpeople is usually "on the job" and MBAs are not often obtained (but this may be changing). Chairpeople are the "face" of the department; therefore, they must attend interdepartmental meetings and functions. Chairpeople are accountable to their department and the public, as well as the hospital chief administrator officers (i.e., CEO, CMO, CQO) and medical college dean [9, 10]. Residency program directors are responsible for all factors affecting the resident's experience, including maintaining ACGME compliance, overseeing resident recruitment/selection/evaluation, and ensuring the welfare of the residents, academic, and otherwise [11]. Residency program directors are accountable to the chair, ACGME, GME office, and residents. The radiology directors and nurse manager duties are somewhat similar. Radiology directors are typically senior RTs responsible for maintaining image quality and regulatory compliance, as well as obtaining/maintaining equipment within a budget. Radiology nurse managers are senior RNs who are responsible for patient and staff safety, regulatory compliance, and staff hiring/training; radiology directors also have these responsibilities, only with respect to the RTs. Of these two administrators, the radiology manager is the one that works closest with the chair/practice director.

Say the word "administrator" to most anybody and you'll get an eyeroll. *Good, solid* administrators are tasked with making difficult, and sometimes unpopular, decisions. They are blamed for things that they can't do anything about and are tasked with implementing departmental changes that were not their idea and they cannot change. Administrators are seen as powerful (because they hire/fire), when, in fact, they are very vulnerable to many groups of people above and below them in the hierarchy, people who don't understand their job complexity but have no problem complaining about it. Political astuteness and a thick skin help management deal with their job stressors, but only to a point. In short, don't aggravate them, and if you must do something that will likely annoy them, be measured about it. Avoid constantly complaining without providing viable solutions and/or otherwise being a valuable departmental contributor, and avoid being selfish about your own needs [9]. An ounce of understanding and diplomacy goes a long way to building administrator relationships. It will be worth it. If management brought you into the department, they can take you out!

References

1. DaCosta JC. Manual of modern surgery. Philadelphia: Saunders; 1898.
2. Earn ARRT Credentials: Primary Eligibility Pathway Requirements. https://www.arrt.org/pages/earn-arrt-credentials/initial-requirements/primary-requirements. Accessed 19 Feb 2024.
3. Earn ARRT Credentials: Postprimary Eligibility Pathway Requirements. https://www.arrt.org/pages/earn-arrt-credentials/initial-requirements/postprimary-requirement. Accessed 19 Feb 2024.
4. ARRT Reference Documents: Examination Content Specifications. https://www.arrt.org/pages/arrt-reference-documents/by-document-type/examination-content-specifications. Accessed 19 Feb 2024.
5. ACGME Program Requirements for Graduate Medical Education in Interventional Radiology, p 24–31. www.acgme.org. 1 July 2022. Accessed 19 Feb 2024.
6. American Board of Radiology. Initial certification for diagnostic radiology. Initial certification. The Exams. www.theabr.com/diagnostic-radiology/initial-certification. 1 Jul 2022. Accessed 19 Feb 2024.
7. NurseJournal. Steps to becoming a registered nurse. https://nursejournal.org/registered-nursing/how-to-become-a-rn/. Accessed 19 Feb 2024.
8. NurseJournal. How to become a nurse practitioner. https://nursejournal.org/nurse-practitioner/how-to-become-a-nphttps://nursejournal.org/registered-nursing/how-to-become-a-rn/. Accessed 19 Feb 2024.

9. Shuman William P, Sahani Dushyant W. Invited commentary. How to take good care of your radiology department chair and why. J Comput Assist Tomogr. 2023;47:680–1. https://doi.org/10.1097/RCT.0000000000001495.

10. Julius Barry. So, you want to become a radiology chair? 2020. https://radsresident.com/2020/03/01/becoming-a-radiology-chair/. Accessed 19 Feb 2024.

11. Mainiero Martha B. Responsibilities of the program director. Acad Radiol. 2003;10(Suppl 1):S16–20.

Chapter 41
Interactions with Industry

Priya Mody

What Is "Industry"?

An industry is a group of companies related to their primary business. The medical industry comprises groups that provide goods and services for patient care. Within radiology specifically, this includes software and artificial intelligence development firms and manufacturers of imaging machines, procedural equipment, and implantable materials. Aside from physicians and other patient care team members, these are components of the healthcare industry that provide the tools for diagnosing and treating the population. Due to the constant advancement of technology, radiology is a field that has developed strong bonds with its industry partners. However, physicians must consider the potential unintended consequences of these interactions on patient care.

Advantages and Disadvantages of Industry Relationships

Manufacturers are a significant funding source for research, quality improvement, and education initiatives [1]. Their support helps advance medical knowledge and allows for technological innovation. However, relationships between industry partners and physicians can lead to the development of unconscious biases. These biases can influence medical decision-making, such as leading physicians to choose one product over another similar one, even if it is not better or appropriate for the patient. In research settings, underlying biases could result in data manipulation or product presentation in a more favorable light.

P. Mody (✉)
Department of Radiology, University of North Carolina at Chapel Hill, Chapel Hill, NC, USA

© The Author(s), under exclusive license to Springer Nature   195
Switzerland AG 2025
J. Shames et al. (eds.), *A Radiologist's Path*,
https://doi.org/10.1007/978-3-031-86882-5_41

It is vital to adhere to professional standards when interacting with vendors to prevent the development of predispositions regarding available products. This is not to say that you cannot develop preferences by testing the available merchandise. However, those preferences should come from personal experience and not financial or nonfinancial returns.

Guidelines for Appropriate Interactions

The American Association of Medical Colleges (AAMC) established a task force that released a report in 2008 on industry funding of medical education [2]. This report directed academic medical centers to institute policies for good contact between industry partners and educational faculty, students, and staff. Several situations are addressed, including receiving gifts, food, or other types of reimbursement, industry-sponsored programs and scholarships, and site access for vendors. In these centers of learning, every attempt should be made to maintain the integrity and objectivity of the academic environment.

The Council for Medical Specialty Societies (CMSS) has published a document entitled "Code for Interactions with Companies," which has been adopted by the governing organizations of many specialties, including the American College of Radiology (ACR) [3]. While this code applies mainly to the interactions of larger organizations with industry, the document defines many terms regarding types of compensation. These are applicable even at an individual level and are helpful to review. Additionally, guidelines are provided for situations such as awarding research funding, creating clinical practice guidelines, society meetings, and advertising (among others).

Many institutions (especially public and academic entities) have in-house policies detailing activities that are and are not permitted concerning industry vendors. These will vary among different educational institutions and private practice groups. Some examples of these activities include:

- Meet and greets with local and regional manufacturer representatives.
- Industry-sponsored dinners introducing new products.
- Training courses with flights and accommodation sponsored by vendors.
- Honorariums for speaking about a specific product to a group of peers.
- Research funding from partners for studying their products.
- Consulting fees for product development.

These policies aim to reduce potential conflicts of interest and preserve our patients' trust that they will be treated according to the highest standards. Becoming familiar with your group's policy regarding appropriate interactions with industry partners is strongly recommended anytime you begin a new position.

Physician Payments Sunshine Act

Official legislation was passed in 2013 to create transparency in financial relationships between physicians and the industry [4]. The act requires reporting "transactions of value" more significant than $10. This refers to monetary compensation and gifts such as honorariums, experiences, or meals. This data is submitted to a database by manufacturers (the Open Payments Program, maintained by the Centers for Medicare and Medicaid Services). Physicians are allowed to review this information annually before it is publicly available. The system is intended to disclose any possible conflicts of interest you may have to the public.

Objective Product Evaluation

As a clinician, you should develop a system for evaluating products objectively when manufacturers present them. Continually educate yourself on the approved and contraindicated uses of clinical tools when they come to market. There may be some trial and error while you assess your options and learn the benefits and pitfalls of similar products. You also want to ensure adequate product support in case maintenance or troubleshooting of a device is required—particularly in purchasing large imaging equipment. Going through a standardized process can decrease the chances of developing an unintended bias toward any specific item. Perry et al. presented one methodical approach that may apply in both public and private settings [5].

No matter what your evaluation protocols are, it is essential to be mindful of the fact that subconscious biases are quickly developed. Industry product representatives are charismatic and friendly, but their goal is, first and foremost, to convince you to purchase their products over others. With this knowledge, you can focus on the data to make the best decision for yourself (or your institution).

References

1. Lewin J, Arend TE. Industry and the profession of medicine: balancing appropriate relationships with the need for innovation. J Vasc Surg. 2011;54(3)
2. Council of Medical Specialty Societies. Code for Interactions with Companies.
3. Association of American Medical Colleges. AAMC Report on Industry Funding of Medical Education.
4. Agrawal S, Brennan N, Budetti P. The sunshine act – effects on physicians. N Engl J Med. 2013;368(22):2054–7.
5. Perry D, Khorsand D, McNeeley M. A radiologist's guide to the industry: a methodical approach to physician-industry relationships in radiology. Curr Probl Diagn Radiol. 2017;46(3):173–6.

Chapter 42
The Faceless Radiologist No More: Interactions with Patients

Robyn G. Roth

The Faceless Radiologist No More: Interactions with Patients

It is often assumed incorrectly that all radiologists have little to no patient interaction and, in some cases, that could not be further from the truth. Part of the beauty of radiology is that you have some control over your level of patient interaction based on your subspecialty choice and work environment. For instance, radiologists who prefer minimal to no patient interaction may seek a teleradiology position working evening hours. Whereas those who enjoy working in a patient-centered clinic may prefer, breast and interventional radiology. The ability to choose your level of patient interaction makes radiology such a desirable field in the long run.

No matter your subspecialty, all radiologists interact regularly with other healthcare professionals, including doctors, technologists, nurses, and schedulers, so interacting with people is unavoidable (apologies if you chose this specialty thinking otherwise).

Radiology Reports

To patients, radiologists are usually faceless names on their "overpriced" imaging reports. Some patients may never read their radiology reports, while others will cling to your every word, especially those waiting to discover if their disease has progressed. Some may google your credentials, often when questioning the accuracy of your interpretation. Now with electronic medical records, radiology reports become immediately available to the patient, often before the referring physician

R. G. Roth (✉)

Department of Radiology, Cooper University Hospital, Camden, NJ, USA

e-mail: roth-robyn@CooperHealth.edu

© The Author(s), under exclusive license to Springer Nature Switzerland AG 2025

J. Shames et al. (eds.), *A Radiologist's Path*,

https://doi.org/10.1007/978-3-031-86882-5_42

has had time to discuss the results. This is an increasing dilemma and deserves its chapter on navigating these complex situations.

Despite the usually behind-the-scenes role that a radiologist might appear to play, a skilled radiologist is an essential part of the team who can make a significant impact on the healthcare journey of an individual. You will learn early on in your career that your words have lots of meaning and may even mean the difference between life and death, surgery, or palliative care.

As you progress in your career and develop a professional reputation, doctors and patients will start to pay more attention to the radiologist interpreting their reports, especially if they had a particularly positive or negative experience. Watch any experienced physician walk into the reading room and immediately seek out the most reputable radiologist, one they can rely on to consistently provide accurate and reliable information to help them distinguish between disease processes. Some radiologists are so talented that they border on pathologists, being able to determine the subtype of renal cell carcinoma based on imaging findings alone. The most incredible day of your radiology career is when physicians come to the reading room to seek you out specifically.

Radiologists' Interactions with the General Public

Most of the general public will have yet to learn what a radiologist does, and many will not even realize you are a doctor. For those who do understand that you are a doctor who interprets images, they will incorrectly assume that you specialize in all imaging, which means that they will frequently ask your opinion on any imaging test they ever have. Your family and friends do not care that you completed your subspecialty training in breast imaging and have not looked at a hip MRI in 15 years; they will still seek out your expertise. While this might seem illogical and somewhat frustrating at times, your knowledge of general radiology is truly an asset to yourself and others that cannot be underemphasized.

Additionally, your knowledge of screening imaging recommendations for the general public will make you extremely popular with friends and family, especially once they turn 40. I can't tell you the number of times I got sidelined at a party and asked, "My mom had premenopausal breast cancer, and I have dense breast tissue; should I be getting a breast MRI?" (The answer is yes!)

Your medical degree and training in radiology may also unlock many doors beyond the reading room. Your unique skill set and expertise will make you highly desirable as a consultant to medical imaging and device companies, technological startups, artificial intelligence, and medical litigators. If interpreting radiology studies is less fulfilling than you hoped, thankfully, there are many different pathways in which you could use your medical expertise.

This is all to say that you have chosen a great specialty that will serve you and others in the future, no matter your level of patient interaction.

Radiologists' Interactions with Patients

As mentioned previously, several subspecialties in radiology are very patient centric, such as breast imaging and interventional radiology. Unfortunately, most patients do not meet a radiologist in person until something is wrong. (Read that again!) This unique role of a radiologist makes interpersonal skills extremely important.

As a breast radiologist, I work daily in a breast imaging center. Most of my patients are women who fear they have breast cancer. They have either been recalled from their mammogram, have a concerning clinical exam finding, or are being followed closely. Either way, they are scared; you can see it in their eyes when you walk through the door.

As a radiologist in this situation, we have a unique opportunity to help people in a very vulnerable state. This is usually our first meeting, and they come to me looking for answers and guidance. I look them in the eye and explain the findings and next steps, which often might be a biopsy. Tears are shed. I comfort them and tell them it will be ok, even though it might be a long road.

I perform the biopsy and give results a few days later, often a breast cancer diagnosis. I ensure they are not driving or sitting in the break room at work. I try my best to be concise and transparent, to say the word "cancer" because anything else does not get through. I assure them that I will help them assemble a fantastic breast cancer team who will take good care of them. I acknowledge that this is overwhelming and encourage them to write down any questions that might arise after we get off the phone. The reality of their diagnosis washes over them. I take my time and give them my phone number, just in case. I tell them it will be a rough year or few, but they will persevere and come out stronger.

In many cases, I am the first doctor someone might see when diagnosed with breast cancer. Before any phone call, I internally acknowledge the gravity of the situation that this person is receiving possibly the worst news of her life. I take the time to look in their chart to see if anyone has discussed the possibility of a cancer diagnosis, or am I pulling the rug out from underneath her? I check any breast specialist notes to ensure there isn't a plan already in place so we're all on the same page. Speaking from personal experience, this extra step is essential and will make you a highly respected member of the breast cancer team.

I usually encounter a patient more than once during their cancer journey and often develop a special bond despite our few unpleasant encounters. The best part of the job is seeing someone a year after their breast cancer diagnosis, usually after they have completed treatment and are returning for their first postoperative mammogram. There is no better feeling than reassuring them that everything looks good and we'll see them in 6–12 months; their sigh of relief and giant hug makes it all worth it.

Beyond the Reading Room: Radiologists in Social Media

Recent studies showed that more than 50 % of Americans ages 18-49 turn to social media (SoMe) for health information, with onethird citing TikTok as their main source of health information, and that number is likely growing [1, 2]. With the rise in social media, many radiologists are stepping out of the darkroom and into the spotlight on social media. Many radiologists (myself included) have successfully turned to social media (#SoMe) to network, educate, collaborate, and advocate. In this section, I will provide an overview of social media use in radiology, including pros and cons, things to consider before starting a social media, lessons learned from my popular breast health social media platform, and tips for anyone interested.

The number of doctors on social media is growing and will likely continue to increase in popularity with the younger generation of doctors. Doctors can reach a more extensive, younger audience by meeting people where they are.

Radiologists may choose to use social media for several reasons, including the following:

- Sharing interesting cases (HIPAA compliant, obviously!)
- Highlighting the role of a radiologist and life outside the office.
- Networking and collaborating with like-minded physicians.
- Educating about important screening recommendations for the general public.
- Combatting medical misinformation.
- Advocating for early detection and insurance coverage.

There are increasing social media channels, which will also likely increase over time. Some of the most popular platforms include Instagram, TikTok, YouTube, Twitter, Facebook, Reddit, and Doximity, to name a few. Each forum has different audiences, pros and cons, and other keys to success (the nuances of which are beyond the scope of this book). It can be daunting to remain active across all platforms, so it's best to focus on 2–3 media when starting.

From my experience, TikTok provides the fastest growth potential, but the vast audience makes it harder to develop a niche. X/Twitter is a great way to connect to other healthcare professionals, with no pictures necessary. Instagram allows you to build a brand and a loyal following, and YouTube is great for educational videos (shorter versions of which can be repurposed for TikTok and Instagram reels).

Consistency is critical with social media; followers will expect consistent content as you grow, so only bite off what you can chew in the beginning. Some content can be shared across multiple platforms; for instance, a video posted on TikTok may also be posted on Instagram, Facebook reels, and YouTube shorts.

Reputable doctors on social media are more integral than ever. With the rise in medical misinformation, mainly stemming from political undertones surrounding the COVID-19 pandemic, medical misinformation on social media is at an all-time high. Social media can effectively combat this misinformation and spread important imaging recommendations to the general public and other healthcare professionals.

Pros and Cons of Social Media

Several pros and cons associated with social media need to be considered before making an online presence, detailed below.

Pros

- **It allows you to share your knowledge and medical training with a larger audience.** Through social media, you can educate directly to other healthcare professionals and the general public about your area of expertise. You can use social media to share essential screening recommendations, highlight interesting cases and procedures (don't forget HIPAA!), showcase new technologies, and document your path to becoming a radiologist. You may even choose to highlight a disease process you are passionate about.
- **The creative outlet allows you to highlight and connect on interests outside the reading room.** Don't pigeonhole yourself just to radiology. You are a multi-faceted being, and this is an opportunity to share what makes you unique! Social media provides an incredible opportunity to highlight your hobbies and connect with those with similar interests (baking, fashion, traveling, mountain climbing, etc.; the more unique, the better!)
- **Provides a means for professional engagement, mentorship, and connection.** There is a growing internet community of social media medical professionals and advocates. Social media broadens your horizons and allows you to connect and collaborate with like-minded and interesting people from all over the world whom you might not have otherwise met. But be warned—this is also a double-edged sword—the internet is forever, so negative online interactions may haunt you in the future.
- **Recruitment tool** (the efficacy of which is surprisingly high!). This is particularly helpful when seeking residency/fellowship positions or job openings. There is an increasing trend on X/Twitter where radiology applicants declare that they are entering the Match, highlight some of their achievements and interests, and hopefully catch the eye of program directors. The same goes for programs looking to fill vacant residency and fellowship programs or groups looking to hire. Social media as a recruitment tool will likely increase over time.
- **Become an advocate.** You may advocate for insurance coverage of particular imaging modalities/procedures, a specific disease process, or your professional interests. Social media allows you to connect or get the attention of people and organizations with similar passions and interests. For instance, breast surgical

oncologists on social media are currently gaining the attention of patients and insurance companies fighting over insurance reimbursement for DIEP flaps.

- **Potential brand partnerships or revenue.** *This cannot/should not be your primary goal to starting a social media account* (read that again). Don't expect Figs to knock at your door because you posted a cute pic in their newest color. The hard truth is that most doctors on social media will not garner a large following, and those that do find success will not achieve it overnight. As the number of healthcare professionals on social media increases, gaining a following is becoming increasingly more complex. Success on social media requires hard work, dedication, and perseverance. It may take years before hitting 1000 followers and many more years to catch the attention of brands willing to send you products or money for your content.

Risks

- **Confidentiality.** It is crucial to remember HIPAA when highlighting a case on social media, particularly when images are being shared. Always de-identify patient information when discussing specifics or showing pictures of an issue.
- **Anyone can find you on social media, including patients, programs, potential programs, and employers.** Social media is the new Google, and your internet personality may precede you. Treat social media like everyone is watching you because they are. Though social media can be a great way to attract patients, it can also work against you. It's important to remember that the internet is forever, and a seemingly innocent comment on another doctor's post may come back to haunt you. Always be professional and treat others with respect, no matter how much you disagree with their point of view.
- **Damage to your professional reputation.** See above.
- **Job security.** Make sure to follow the social media policies and procedures set forth by your institution. They will likely ask you to refrain from posting at work and keep your hospital branding out.
- **Legal issues.** For all of the reasons above, putting yourself on social media puts you at risk for potential legal trouble you might not have otherwise encountered. Also, consider working on an intellectual property contract with your institution before your account is successful or has any monetary value. Despite the possibility of legal issues, several pros outweigh the possibility of legal trouble. Play by the above rules to set yourself up for success.

My Success

Over 40,000 of my closest internet friends call me @theboobiedocs, my popular social media account that discusses breast cancer in a fun and educational way. Through social media success, I have launched a successful Podcast, "The Girlfriend's Guide to Breast Cancer," to help those navigating a breast cancer diagnosis, was on the cover of my local newspaper, and I have had several television appearances, including kicking off Breast Cancer Awareness Month on *Today with Hoda and Jenna* in October 2021. I became a Figs ambassador in 2022 and have been invited to give several lectures to local and national cancer organizations,

My social media success did not happen overnight. I officially joined Instagram in October 2018 with the handle @drrobynroth (genius, I know!). After a few awkward selfies in front of the workstation, I struggled to find my voice and posted sparingly over the next 2 years. One late night while breastfeeding my third child during the COVID-19 pandemic and realizing I was surrounded by breasts all day, I had my "aha!" moment. I changed the name to @theboobiedocs in 2020, the "-s" reflecting my best friend/colleague who ultimately left social media. "We are working moms, best friends, and breast cancer advocates," I explained. I realized I could talk directly to young women like myself to discuss essential but controversial breast cancer screening recommendations and connect with people affected by breast cancer. Once I found my voice, everything fell into place; the content was endless, and the growth was exponential.

Social media has given me a purpose and passion outside the reading room. It has made my career much more fulfilling than it would have been otherwise and allows me to combine my love for writing and early breast cancer detection and connect with people worldwide.

Here's my best advice for any radiologist looking to venture into social media.

1. **Find your voice. Incorporate your personality and passions.** Also, when choosing a handle, think long term. It is important to remember that you probably will not be at your current institution forever, so unless. Unless you are running a hospital-approved social media account (which usually has more hurdles and has to be approved by the administration), leave your institution's name out of your social media handle.
2. **Learn your audience.** Are you looking to connect with patients, radiologists, or neither? Tailor your posts accordingly.
3. **Don't be afraid to put yourself out there.** Document your wins and your losses. The more transparent and open you are, the more likely you are to develop an engaged audience and keep their attention.
4. **Be active across all platforms.** Content from one social media platform can be tweaked to fit other platforms. For instance, a TikTok may be cross-posted to Instagram, Facebook Reels, and YouTube shorts. Consistency is key. Aim to post at least 2–3 times a week to keep your audience engaged and wanting more.
5. **Have fun and be authentic.** Social media is a hobby long before it becomes part of your career. Have fun, be yourself, and you never know the doors that may open up or the people you might connect with.

References

1. Wang X, Cohen RA. Health information technology use among Overview adults: United States, July–December 2022. NCHS Data Brief, no 482. Hyattsville, MD: National Center for Health Statistics. 2023. https://dx.doi.org/10.15620/cdc:133700.
2. SoMe in Healthcare Statistics 2024 By data, insights, Engagement. Accessed 7/2/24 https://media.market.us/social-media-in-healthcare-statistics/.

Chapter 43
Professionalism in Radiology Residency and Beyond

Theresa Kaufman

Beyond clinical expectations of excellence, what you will be known for, in a nutshell, is your professionalism. The term "professionalism" is indistinct. It has many definitions and encompasses many attributes. Merriam-Webster defines it as "the conduct, aims, or qualities that characterize or mark a profession or a professional person." The American Board of Internal Medicine's Physician Charter of Medical Professionalism characterized professionalism as the basis of medicine's contract with society and set forth fundamental principles and responsibilities which apply to all physicians [1]. While these intricacies go beyond the scope of this chapter, it is essential to note that professionalism is a set of traits and behaviors that affects the daily practice of all radiologists and will be assessed repeatedly over the course of training. It is one of the six core competencies set forth by the Accreditation Council for Graduate Medical Education (ACGME), assessed continuously during residency, and tested on the Noninterpretive Skills section of the Radiology Core Examination [2–4]. Many aspects of your professionalism may already be engrained in who you are. Still, it is an entity that can be molded over time through positive and negative reinforcement with our interactions with others and learned by the example of our mentors. In this chapter, we will review some practical pearls and basic expectations of professionalism that will help you succeed in residency and beyond.

T. Kaufman (✉)
Department of Radiology, Thomas Jefferson University Hospitals, Philadelphia, PA, USA
e-mail: Theresa.kaufman@jefferson.edu

J. Shames et al. (eds.), *A Radiologist's Path*,
https://doi.org/10.1007/978-3-031-86882-5_43

The Work: Putting the Profession Into "Professionalism"

For residents, trainees' expectations will vary depending on PGY level and from program to program, but how you handle yourself will speak volumes about who you are as a professional. Remember, residency is a job. You are there to learn and are being paid to do so while working in a predominantly apprenticeship-style environment to become the best-practicing radiologist you can be.

Be punctual. Stay until the end of the workday. Take every case as a learning opportunity. Come prepared having read and with an open mind to ask questions so you can continuously improve and expand your knowledge, no matter what phase in training. If there is some downtime, choosing to use it to read an article rather than surf the web on the side computer will go a long way, and your attendings will notice (whether you think they do or not—it is their job to see details!). Incorporate the feedback given to you. By doing so, you will demonstrate your commitment to your own education and clinical competence and the desire to improve the quality of care for your patients. If you don't know what is expected of you, ask.

The Patients

Radiologists are often called the "doctor's doctor," referring to the service we provide to clinicians and how we can help them manage their patients by interpreting imaging studies. We must also remember that a person is behind those images, and you are also *their* doctor. This may be easier in specific subspecialties where there is more direct patient contact, and delivering bad news and obtaining informed consent are additional ways to practice and refine our professional behavior. The art of communicating with patients requires practice, but even for those subspecialties where there is rare direct patient care, if we first and foremost remember that there is a person behind the images, the commitment as a physician to place our patients' interests first becomes nature rather than a responsibility.

Communication

While some still think of radiologists as physicians who seek to sit in a dark room away from society, we interact with people all day. If lists are long and work is overwhelming, interruptions to field consults and phone calls for protocols can be stressful while attempting to focus on image interpretation. Whether interacting with technologists, nurses, administrative support staff, referring clinicians, trainees, or each other, try to remain patient—be a good citizen, help each other out, and treat everyone with respect.

Furthermore, we communicate with referring clinicians and our patients most frequently through our reports. The images and our interpretations are enduring material. It is important to get the facts correct and accurate information. Templates and dictation software help with efficiency but are only valuable if right. Proofread—practicing doing so during training will make it easier to do as second nature when alone. In today's age of the twenty-first Century Cures Act, which allows patients immediate access to results, our reports and communication efforts may be scrutinized immediately by the patients themselves.

Of course, we are all human beings, and mistakes can happen. If you make a mistake, own up to it. This goes beyond reports—accept that you could be better and know when to ask questions and when to ask for help. If you don't see an answer, always try your best but don't pretend or make things up.

What about non-work-related communication? We spend most of our waking hours at work, and our coworkers become friends. This can blur the lines of friendly versus professional communication. When in doubt, err on the side of caution. Keep jokes clean, keep your hands to yourself, and know your audience.

Challenges

As a trainee, each day may present a challenge as you attempt to be a chameleon, adjusting to variations in read-out sessions, search patterns, reporting styles, and approach to procedures depending on differing attendings. Generally, try to ensure that your reports reflect your discussion with your attending. What to do if you disagree? It is ok to have a difference in opinion. Approach each case courteously and directly, and discuss your concerns with the attending radiologist. Most of the time, they will either agree with your assessment or explain why they feel their initial assessment is correct so that you understand their evidence-based point of view. Ultimately, they are the final say, but if you feel strongly about your opinion, seek advice from a mentor on how to proceed.

Do you have issues with certain aspects of your program? Every program has ways to improve. Figure out modifiable topics important to you and find avenues to provide constructive criticism so that the program can make measurable progress to help your success and that of your peers.

As a more significant issue, there may be generational differences in professional values between you as a trainee or early career radiologist and those who have come before you. Additionally, in this post-pandemic era, physicians may be confronted with competing obligations to our families, patients, and each other. Open lines of communication with each other will be important moving forward as we work together through these challenges.

Bottom Line

Though many of the pearls presented in this chapter may sound straightforward, they can be challenging to remember when faced with strong personalities and in the setting of long lists and time pressures. As physicians, our ultimate goal is quality patient care. The path we choose to take to get there is affected by our professionalism, encompassing our clinical proficiency and day-to-day interactions with all of those we encounter.

References

1. American Board of Internal Medicine Foundation. Medical professionalism in the new millennium: the physician charter. American Board of Internal Medicine Foundation Website. https://abimfoundation.org/what-we-do/medicalprofessionalism-and-the-physician-charter/physician-charter.
2. American College of Radiology Bylaws Code of Ethics. American College of Radiology website. https://www.acr.org/-/media/ACR/Files/Governance/Bylaws.pdf.
3. The Accreditation Council for Graduate Medical Education. Diagnostic radiology milestones. https://www.acgme.org/globalassets/pdfs/milestones/diagnosticradiologymilestones.pdf.
4. American Board of Radiology. Noninterpretive skills study guide. https://www.theabr.org/wp-content/uploads/2022/04/2022-NIS-Study-Guide-v2.pdf.

Part IV
Long Term Goals and Planning

Chapter 44
Board Exams

Anne Kathryn Misiura

* In January 2023, the ABR provisionally approved a new oral certifying exam to replace the written certifying exam. In April 2023 the following announcement was made: "Beginning in calendar year 2028 and first applying to DR residents completing training in June 2027 (entering their R1 year in July 2023), the certifying exam for DR will be the new DR Oral Exam. From that point on, a candidate's first opportunity to take the new DR Oral Exam will be the calendar year following completion of their DR residency. All DR candidates taking the DR Certifying Exam after 2027 will be required to take the new DR Oral Exam regardless of when they completed residency training. We anticipate having two exam administrations per year." https://www.theabr.org/announcements/new-diagnostic-radiology-oral-exam. Please refer to the ABR website for information regarding the new oral examination format. The following information is in regard to the "old" written certifying exam that will be available until 2027.

The Certifying Exam (CE) is the final step in board certification. Congratulations, this exam is straightforward, tailored to your expertise, and currently administered remotely (sorry if you were very excited to go to Arizona). There is no reported pass rate data from the ABR, but nobody on the internet has ever self-reported failing. Take that for what you will.

To qualify, you must have passed the Qualifying (Core) Exam, usually administered at the end of your third year of radiology residency (R3). No earlier than 12 months after completing residency, you'll be invited to register for the CE, generally taken 15 months after completing residency (or three months after fellowship). Currently, it is only offered once per year. Additional qualifying information is provided in Table 44.1 [1].

A. K. Misiura (✉)
Department of Radiology, Thomas Jefferson University Hospital, Philadelphia, PA, USA
e-mail: anne.misiura@jefferson.edu

© The Author(s), under exclusive license to Springer Nature Switzerland AG 2025
J. Shames et al. (eds.), *A Radiologist's Path*,
https://doi.org/10.1007/978-3-031-86882-5_44

Table 44.1 Requirements to take Certifying Exam (CE)

Be current with all ABR fees and pay all exam fees 60 days before the date of the exam
Hold an active state or provincial (Canadian) medical license
Be board eligible
Have a functional application with the ABR
Complete DR residency or DR IMG plan and clinical year of training requirements
Pass the Qualifying (Core) Exam
Meet the minimum waiting period after training
A 12-month waiting period is required after residency before taking the exam for the standard DR certification pathway
There is no waiting period after training has been successfully completed for IMGs in the Alternate Pathway or those with ABNM certification.

Seven and a half hours are allocated for the one-day CE exam, which consists of 298 questions. There are four modules: the required Essentials of Diagnostic Radiology module and three modules of your choosing. You may choose from general radiology, breast, cardiac, gastrointestinal, musculoskeletal, neuroradiology, nuclear, pediatric, thoracic, ultrasound, genitourinary, and vascular and interventional radiology. You may choose 1, 2, or 3 of the same module. For example, you may select three neuroradiology modules if you've completed a neuroradiology fellowship. You may choose gastrointestinal, genitourinary, and ultrasound if you've completed an abdominal fellowship. The caveat is that if you choose the same module twice or three times, the second and third module questions are considered "advanced" instead of "basic." You should check with recent fellows in your division about their previous choices.

The Essentials of Diagnostic Radiology module is appropriately named, containing content any radiologist should know. For example, even if I read abdominal imaging only, I should still recognize different types of head bleeds on CT. This module also contains questions from the Noninterpretive Skills document provided by the ABR, including questions on ethics, professionalism, error prevention, and other aspects of practice [2].

Also included throughout the exam are physics questions and Radioisotope Safety Content (RISC) questions. If you've submitted appropriate documentation during residency and received a passing score on the RISC questions, you'll be given authorized user-eligible (AU-E) status. The RISC result allegedly does not affect the pass results for the Certifying Exam. You cannot opt out of the RISC questions. Pediatric questions are also included in all sections, so don't assume "adult-only" questions if you don't choose the pediatric section.

For more detailed exam content, I refer you to the ABR website.

So how do you study? Note that I have no financial or otherwise relationship with any specific resources mentioned.

Most people use the BoardVitals question bank in their free time for a few weeks before the exam and do not take time off for dedicated study. The CE does not require the intense studying that the Qualifying Core Exam did, but it would behoove you to take it seriously. Don't be an outlier. Subspecialty review books are often used. Check with your fellowship programs or any recently graduates if they have old copies you can borrow. A common study tool for the physics and RISC questions is the e-book Radiology Simplified, available on iTunes [3]. BoardVitals also offers questions in these categories.

For the NIS section, commonly, one would download the ABR-provided document for review on the plane ride down to the exam to keep it fresh. Several YouTube videos now review the content if you prefer an audiovisual format. While these topics may seem straightforward, the language may confuse you (even if you check the document), so don't disregard this content.

Be sure to request time off to take the exam, which you'll most likely take while employed.

You are considered "board eligible" until you pass the exam. If you do not pass the exam within six years from the end of your training, you'll have to take another year of training at an ACGME-accredited program to reenter the certification process.

Exam results as pass/fail only, no scoring, are available approximately one month after the exam.

Anecdotally, no one I talked to immediately following the exam was ever confident they passed; on the contrary, they were either sure they failed or indifferent about it. And they all passed, as expected. So, get on with it and don't stress.

References

1. Prerequisites and Registration [Internet]. The American Board of Radiology. 2022 [cited 2023Feb22]. https://www.theabr.org/diagnostic-radiology/initial-certification/certifying-exam/prerequisites-registration
2. 2022 Noninterpretive Skills – The American Board of Radiology [Internet]. [cited 2023Feb22]. https://www.theabr.org/wp-content/uploads/2022/04/2022-NIS-Study-Guide-v2.pdf
3. Srinivasan L, Park J. Radiology simplified. Transcend Review; 2021.

Chapter 45
Learning New Procedures

Priya Mody

The Learning Process

Completion of training is not the end of learning in medicine. The first few months to years following graduation especially are a period of rapid and significant growth for an early career physician. You may encounter situations in practice that require you to expand your procedural skill set beyond what you learned as a resident. However, unlike in training, resources to build those skills may not be readily accessible [1]. You will have to determine the best way to gain this new knowledge to provide competent care to your patients.

In addition to learning these new skills, you must know how to improve on them. Repetition is naturally important to build confidence and gain experience. Asking for and accepting feedback from other skilled practitioners is crucial to improving your newly acquired skills [2]. You will also need to keep up with changes in guidelines or new developments by continuing to read current literature or attending conferences.

Self-Education

As medical trainees, we are taught to improve our knowledge gaps by self-guided learning. We read textbooks and journals and, in the age of technology, watch educational webinars and video tutorials. Self-education is a viable method to learn variations of or troubleshoot procedures you already know. For example, you may use the manufacturer's guide and/or training video learn to use a biopsy needle

P. Mody (✉)
Department of Radiology, University of North Carolina at Chapel Hill, Chapel Hill, NC, USA

J. Shames et al. (eds.), *A Radiologist's Path*,
https://doi.org/10.1007/978-3-031-86882-5_45

different from the one you trained with in residency. This method is not recommended for more complex procedures or ones you are completely inexperienced with.

Mentorship

If your colleagues are already performing a procedure in practice, the easiest way to learn it is to be mentored by them. This is most similar to the way you learned during training and has several benefits. First, you will be taught the same method used by others in the group, allowing for consistency among physicians. Additionally, someone can talk you through troubleshooting and improving technique over time. Even if you encounter a difficult situation several months after learning the procedure, you can still ask for assistance from a partner. Lastly, this method builds trust and encourages collaboration between you and your colleagues, enhancing your overall work environment.

Mentorship can also come from former attendings and colleagues. Most teaching faculty enjoy hearing from prior trainees and are more than happy to offer over-the-phone guidance for new or difficult cases. By utilizing them as a resource, you will start your career with multiple "go-to" people for the various types of procedures you will be doing. Additionally, as you and your colleagues go your separate ways, you may all learn different methods of approaching a problem or start using different devices. Sharing any newfound knowledge and experiences as a group can be beneficial to all of you.

Proctoring

If you are trying to incorporate a new procedure into your practice that is not already performed by someone in your group, you may benefit from a proctor. This is someone who comes in from outside your department or institution to teach a specific procedure or technique. They are often sponsored by industry - to demonstrate usage of a new device, for example. The proctor will spend a few hours to a couple days walking you through the process and ensuring you are comfortable with it. While traditionally proctoring is done in person, teleproctoring has increased in popularity following the COVID-19 pandemic and can be a valuable resource if you are practicing in a rural area.

CME Courses

Formal workshops or courses may be required to learn more complex or newly developed procedures (e.g., stroke interventions, kyphoplasty, ablation, etc.). If you are interested in building your practice to include procedures you have limited or no prior experience with, a dedicated course can ensure that you learn the correct technique and troubleshooting methods to provide safe care. The cost of attending these courses may be covered by your CME stipend, if you have one, so be aware of this or any other educational resources offered in your contract. Additionally, these are a good source of CME for maintenance of certification.

References

1. White B. Growing as a new radiology attending. Ben White | Medicine & Miscellany. 2024, March 6. https://www.benwhite.com/radiology/growing-as-a-new-attending/
2. White B. Crowdsourced advice for being a young radiology attending. Ben White | Medicine & Miscellany. 2023, November 2. https://www.benwhite.com/radiology/crowdsourced-advice-on-being-a-young-radiology-attending/

Chapter 46
Research

Tessa S. Cook

Introduction

The term "research" may conjure up a vision of bench lab work, basic science experiments, pipettes, and microscopic samples. However, research in radiology can be very broadly defined. It spans the gamut from basic science work with cells and animals to the development of artificial intelligence algorithms with sophisticated computing hardware. In this chapter, we consider the different types of research performed in radiology, how research results can be disseminated, and sources of funding for research.

Types of Research in Radiology

There are many types of research in radiology. These include the following:

- Basic science.
- Clinical.
- Clinical trials.
- Quality improvement.
- Innovation.
- Practice transformation.

T. S. Cook (✉)
Department of Radiology, Perelman School of Medicine at the University of Pennsylvania, Philadelphia, PA, USA
e-mail: tessa.cook@pennmedicine.upenn.edu

© The Author(s), under exclusive license to Springer Nature Switzerland AG 2025
J. Shames et al. (eds.), *A Radiologist's Path*,
https://doi.org/10.1007/978-3-031-86882-5_46

Basic science research in radiology is particularly common with the development of radiotracers for nuclear medicine as well as catheter-directed therapies for oncology in interventional radiology. Both these fields involve bench work as well as cellular and animal research. The development of novel image reconstruction and processing techniques is another common area of basic science research. Radiomics, which involves understanding higher-order imaging features and their relationship to diagnosis and treatment planning, is a popular subfield of basic science research in radiology.

Clinical research in radiology can take a variety of forms. It can involve retrospective research, which focuses on the analysis of patients with a certain diagnosis being evaluated with a particular imaging modality or a comparison of the impact of different imaging modalities. It can also involve prospective research that resembles clinical trials to evaluate a new modality or imaging technique compared to usual care. **Comparative effectiveness research** compares two different real-world pathways for management and treatment and, in radiology, often includes a comparison of different modalities for the evaluation of disease [1].

Clinical trials in radiology can be prospective or retrospective to analyze new imaging modalities, analysis techniques, or treatment pathways [2]. There are multiple barriers radiologists might face in conducting clinical trials, including insufficient training, sufficient time to manage trials, and insufficient funding.

Quality improvement is a critical component of any radiology department or practice. It improves the performance and processes related to imaging care and spans the spectrum from the very first interaction a patient has with radiology (e.g., registration, scheduling, etc.) to image interpretation, results communication, and follow-up monitoring [3]. Quality improvement research often follows a plan-do-study-act (PDSA) cycle or other related paradigm for continuous evaluation and improvement of a process within a department or practice.

Innovation and practice transformation are nontraditional research avenues that focus on existing clinical practice and explore opportunities to improve both clinician and patient experience and outcomes [4]. Innovation seeks to develop novel approaches to care delivery that may use disruptive technologies adapted from other industries. Practice transformation similarly seeks to explore new care paradigms that might not necessarily involve new technologies but rather new approaches to how radiologists and patients interact with existing systems. A unique aspect of these types of research is the potential for rapid validation cycles, where a small change is made and its impact is assessed for a short period of time (e.g., 1–2 weeks). Based on the observations made, a new change is implemented, and a new cycle begins. A series of rapid validation cycles can be performed to incrementally assess a larger intervention.

Dissemination of Research

An important aspect of research is the dissemination of results to the larger medical and scientific communities. This is typically accomplished by publications in the peer-reviewed literature, although there are increasingly alternative avenues for sharing scientific explorations and results.

Presentation of research results at a scientific meeting may precede a full manuscript in the literature. This is often an avenue that radiologists and trainees can more easily pursue at all levels. It gives presenters the opportunity to get real-time feedback on their work from an audience of peers. This feedback can be used to inform the way a manuscript is written or also influence plans for future work.

Historically, most scientific papers were published in subscription-only journals after double-blinded peer review (where neither the authors nor the reviewers knew each other's identities). Now, there are journals that offer single-blinded or fully unblinded peer review. In addition, more journals are offering either a subscription or open-access option; in the latter, authors support the cost of publication and dissemination through article processing charges (APCs). Some journals are entirely open access.

More recently, preprint servers (such as http://www.arxiv.org and http://www.medrxiv.org) have become very popular, both as a means for scientists and researchers to freely disseminate their work to a large audience, as well as for authors to get feedback on their papers before submission to a peer-reviewed journal [5]. Although the feedback can be valuable, some journals do not accept papers that have been posted to a preprint server, so authors should consider the risks and benefits of posting their work in advance of submission for peer review.

Research dissemination via social media has also become increasingly popular. Subscription journals often send authors time-limited links to post online to share their work soon after publication. Links to open-access publications and preprint servers are easy to share. This fosters discussion with the larger community about new scientific developments. Authors can also share their work via blog posts; however, these are rarely, if ever, peer reviewed. Nevertheless, they can potentially reach a wider audience than the subscribers to a particular journal.

Grant Funding

Depending on the type of research being performed, radiologists often seek grant funding to support their time away from the clinical service to conduct the work. There are a wide variety of funding sources available to radiologists. The one that most commonly comes to mind is grant funding through the National Institutes of Health (NIH). There are many different levels of funding available through the NIH and its multiple institutes to support investigators at all career levels, preliminary research, and research with preliminary supporting data. Obtaining NIH grant funding can be challenging due to limited funds availability, which is often dictated by Congress, and the number of scientists competing for this limited resource.

Professional societies also offer smaller grants that address areas of scientific study related to their subspecialty focus. These can be more easily accessible to early career scientists and trainees. Although trainees may not need funding to protect their time away from clinical service, it can establish them as qualified early-career investigators and is beneficial to their departments. It can also provide support for scanner time, other resources with a cost attached, or even incentives to patients.

Foundation grants are also a popular option for small grants focused on a particular disease process. These are often an untapped and poorly documented resource that radiologists will have to creatively seek out. They are often also more accessible to early-career radiologists and trainees.

Intramural funds—funding available within a university or academic hospital—may also be an option. These are typically small awards intended to help researchers get preliminary data to support an extramural funding application. Nevertheless, as a starting point, they can be a valuable starting point for new projects and early-career radiologists or those just getting started in research.

As with any grant funding, it is important to craft a project proposal that can realistically be completed with the provided funding and the time it supports. Some funding organizations will provide no-cost extensions (NCEs) which allow researchers additional time to complete the proposed work without additional funding. However, others require strict adherence to the proposed timeline, and not being able to complete the work in the proposed time may jeopardize the success of future applications.

References

1. Pandharipande PV, Gazelle GS. Comparative effectiveness research: what it means for radiology. Radiology. 2009;253(3):600–5.
2. Alvin MD, Moshiri M, Bluemke DA. Prospective clinical trials: 10-year trends in radiology. Radiology. 2020;295(1):1–2.
3. Hoang JK, Menard AR. Innovation in radiology: three-step process to increasing innovation. J Am Coll Rad. 2021;18(3B):514–6.
4. Kruskal JB, Eisenberg R, Sosna J, Yam CS, Kruskal JD, Boiselle PM. Quality improvement in radiology: basic principles and tools required to achieve success. Radiographics. 2011;31(6):1499–509.
5. Flanagin A, Fontanarosa PB, Bauchner H. Preprints involving medical research – do the benefits outweigh the challenges? JAMA. 2020;324(18):1840–3.

Chapter 47
You Can't Spell Radiology Without AI

Tessa S. Cook and Satvik Tripathi

Introduction

Since late 2016, there has been a great deal of buzz about artificial intelligence (AI) in medical imaging, particularly in radiology. The success of the ImageNet challenge a few years earlier demonstrated the power of deep learning, a form of AI, in identifying characteristics of images [1]. Although ImageNet jumpstarted the focus on pixel-based AI in radiology, there are also several non-pixel-based use cases that would benefit from AI [2]. In this chapter, we provide a high-level introduction to AI, discuss opportunities for radiology AI but also concerns, and consider how radiologists can introduce AI into their practices and what our patients currently think about it. Finally, we briefly highlight the current state of the art, acknowledging that this technology is developing rapidly and that techniques and tools discussed in this section may be mainstream or obsolete at some point after this chapter is published.

What Is AI?

The terms "artificial intelligence" and "machine learning" are often used interchangeably or in combination. But what do they actually mean [3]? Figure 47.1 summarizes the various terms and their relationships.

Artificial intelligence describes the field of computer science that studies how computers can mimic human intelligence. Machine learning (ML) is a subset of artificial intelligence, which allows computers to learn without explicitly being programmed.

T. S. Cook (✉) · S. Tripathi
Department of Radiology, Perelman School of Medicine at the University of Pennsylvania, Philadelphia, PA, USA
e-mail: tessa.cook@pennmedicine.upenn.edu

© The Author(s), under exclusive license to Springer Nature Switzerland AG 2025
J. Shames et al. (eds.), *A Radiologist's Path*,
https://doi.org/10.1007/978-3-031-86882-5_47

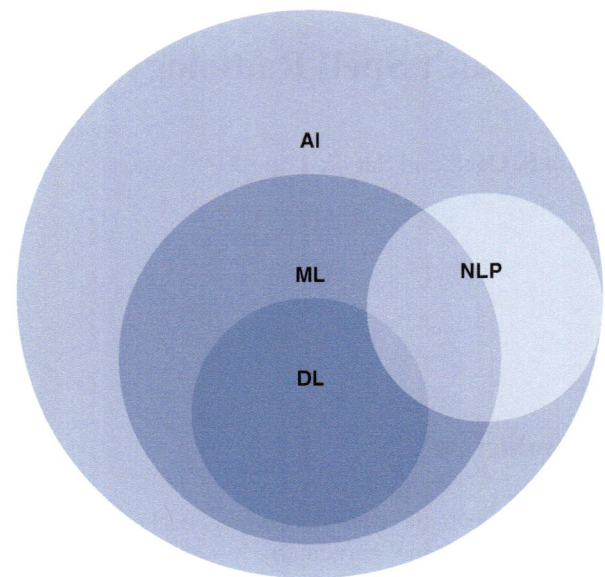

ML includes but is not limited to a variety of neural network-based algorithms. Deep learning (DL), in turn, is a subset of machine learning, which refers to the use of sophisticated neural networks with multiple layers for ML. Natural language processing (NLP), which refers to computer processing of text specifically, overlaps AI, ML, and DL.

AI in radiology most commonly relies on deep learning algorithms that build on architectures originally developed in the 1950s. These techniques are more powerful today, thanks to advances in computing hardware, notably the development of graphical processing units (GPUs), availability of cloud computing, and low cost of memory and storage media. Additionally, there are numerous freely available educational resources that have made it possible for anyone with a GPU and some data to train an AI model, i.e., expose an algorithm to data and develop an AI tool for a particular use case. However, not all these models are instantly ready for clinical use, despite the accessibility of the technology.

Opportunities for AI in Radiology

There are many potential use cases for AI in radiology, spanning pixel-based, and non-pixel-based applications. Pixel-based use cases are likely the most numerous, given the nature of diagnostic and interventional radiology. These tasks primarily represent detecting findings, abnormalities, or entire organs (i.e., segmentation). They can also spawn other steps in the clinical workflow, such as worklist triage, population of the radiology report with measurements or labels, or messages to clinicians within or outside radiology.

For example, AI that looks for intracranial hemorrhage or large vessel occlusion (LVO) can send an electronic alert to a diagnostic radiologist to confirm the diagnosis, as well as to an interventional neuroradiologist or neurosurgeon who could act on the information. Similarly, AI for other critical findings, such as tension pneumothorax, aortic dissection, or acute pulmonary embolism, could alert the interpreting radiologist by flagging an exam on the worklist or moving it to the top. Particularly for practices in which off-hours coverage is slower than daytime coverage, this could improve outcomes for patients.

AI that segments and analyzes organs could play a role in opportunistic screening. For example, segmentation and analysis of the fat content of the liver on CT could assist in earlier diagnosis of metabolic dysfunction–associated steatotic liver disease (MASLD). Analysis of coronary calcium burden on any CT that includes the heart may identify patients sooner who could benefit from referral to a cardiologist for cardiovascular risk factor modification.

Image acquisition can also benefit from AI [4]. Techniques to increase signal to noise, decrease artifacts, optimize scan times, decrease radiation exposure, and reduce or eliminate the need for intravenous contrast can improve image acquisition in the short term but, ideally, improve patient outcomes in the long term.

Non-pixel-based AI is applied to data with radiology other than images, notably radiology reports, utilization data, and scheduling across a department or practice. Radiology reports can be analyzed to identify critical and noncritical actionable findings and alert relevant clinicians. For example, follow-up recommendations could automatically be detected and alerts sent to both referring physicians and, if appropriate, patients, to remind them of the need for further workup. AI could also be used to produce radiology reports tailored to recipients, for example, for referring physicians, specialists, and even patients. With the rise of generative AI models, non-pixel data can be harnessed even more, as discussed in the chapter later.

Analysis of utilization rates could help practices adjust staffing needs accordingly, to optimize exam volumes across available scanners and minimize patient wait times. This type of demand forecasting could be used to dynamically schedule technologists, radiologists, and other members of the radiology team [5].

Concerns About AI in Radiology

For as many opportunities as there are for AI to improve care delivery in radiology, there are also concerns that warrant attention.

Patient privacy and data security must always be a primary consideration. Data are needed to effectively train and test new AI models, and thanks to the AI boom, imaging data have been commoditized. As radiologists, we should take responsibility for appropriately safeguarding our patients' data whenever it is shared or exchanged, whether for research or commercial product development. This includes adherence to the Health Insurance Portability and Accountability Act (HIPAA) Privacy Rule that governs de-identification of patient data.

AI is unlike other software currently used in the clinical workflow in that its performance can degrade over time. This is often referred to as "drift." It ultimately occurs because the input data to the model begins to vary sufficiently from the data used during training. This can be because a practice updates their scanning equipment, changes their imaging protocols, begins performing new procedures, or begins taking care of patients with different characteristics to those represented in the training data. As a result, it is important to carefully monitor AI solutions once they are deployed in the clinical workflow, so that eventual drift is detected before it can potentially harm patients.

Automation bias and algorithm aversion are related concepts that address clinicians' interactions with and trust of AI. Automation bias occurs when the human expert defers to the output from the AI, while algorithm aversion occurs when the human expert dismisses the AI output in favor of their own experience and beliefs. Neither is an ideal situation, as both can result in unnecessary errors that may ultimately harm patients. Radiologists using AI should be mindful of the risks of both as they train and practice.

Getting Started with AI in Your Practice

When getting started with AI in your practice, it is important to think about use cases that may be helpful. These may exist in the form of inefficiencies or pain points in the radiologists' workflow, opportunities to introduce new services to patients or referring clinicians, or instances where the potential for human error could be decreased. Regardless of the use case, it is important to identify the relevant stakeholders before the decision-making process begins. These individuals may not all exist within a radiology department or practice; consider referring clinicians who may be affected and should be included in the conversation. Also include patients whose views on AI in their care should be heard and considered.

In some instances, practices may choose to build their own AI solutions instead of purchasing commercially available solutions. This may be because an appropriate solution is not yet available for purchase but does require the practice to have the necessary technical expertise to develop a solution, as well as the resources to maintain and oversee the tool once it is deployed clinically.

Regardless of the build vs. buy question, every radiology practice needs appropriate AI governance [6]. This includes a plan for AI selection, evaluation, deployment, and monitoring. The relevant stakeholders, who may differ for each AI being considered, should be convened early and involved in the process. Necessary human, technical, and financial resources should be designated and procured, and project management is essential. Practices may even develop an AI strategic plan to more effectively execute their vision [7].

Who Pays for AI?

There have been some paradigms for reimbursement of AI in medical imaging [8]. This has been pioneered with a Current Procedural Terminology (CPT) billing code for the diagnosis of diabetic retinopathy using AI. The New Technology Add-On

Payment (NTAP) supported the first 3 years of a handful of tools to diagnose LVO on CT angiography of the head.

Reimbursement for AI in medical imaging continues to evolve [9]. Although a handful of CPT codes now exist, the cost of most AI tools is still covered by hospitals or radiology practices. This may change in the future as payment models evolve and payors begin to cover more use cases. In the meantime, however, this is also impeding the dissemination of this technology across the field. In addition, it may unnecessarily exacerbate health disparities by limiting AI-augmented diagnosis to patients whose insurance covers this advanced technology.

What Do Patients Think About AI?

One stakeholder group that is often left out of conversations regarding AI is our patients. In a small survey about AI in medicine, patients expressed that AI could play a useful role, such as by providing a second opinion or helping a physician prepare for a patient visit [10]. However, they also expressed concerns about the lack of empathy associated with the technology and the risks of cybersecurity and inaccuracy.

A Pew Research Center survey asked more than 11,000 adults in the United States their opinions on AI in health and medicine [11]. They found that 39% of respondents would feel comfortable if AI were used in their care and that only 38% thought it would improve outcomes for patients. Most respondents felt AI would be adopted in healthcare more quickly than it should be. Approximately half of respondents who thought there was bias in healthcare felt that AI would decrease it.

One patient's perspective on the potential role AI could play in his care is somewhat optimistic [12]. He suggests the possibility that AI could generate tailored reports for both referring physicians and patients and caregivers, without increasing the radiologist's workload. This could, in turn, improve communication between patients, their caregivers, and referring physicians, without compromising the human connection that many patients desire.

The Generation of Generative AI

Generative artificial intelligence (GenAI), particularly large language models (LLMs), is rapidly redefining the radiology landscape by enabling machines to understand and generate medical language with remarkable fluency. These models, such as GPT-4, Llama, and Gemini, are trained on massive datasets that include general and biomedical literature, allowing them to perform complex language tasks like clinical summarization, translation of radiology findings, diagnostic question answering, and structured report generation (Fig. 47.2) [13].

In radiology, LLMs are being applied to generate full-length imaging reports from structured data or voice dictation, often reducing reporting time and improving consistency. They also offer promising capabilities in translating technical radiology terminology into lay-friendly language, helping bridge the communication gap between radiologists and patients, which is increasingly important in value-based care models. Some systems are already integrating LLMs to act as intelligent clinical assistants—responding to queries such as "What is the follow-up for a 6 mm lung nodule in a patient who smokes?" or providing evidence-informed recommendations based on radiology guidelines and literature. In educational settings, generative AI has been used to simulate oral board exams, quiz radiology residents, and create interactive learning environments tailored to the learner's level of expertise.

Recent research has demonstrated that domain-specific models like Radiology-GPT outperform general-purpose LLMs in radiology-specific tasks, particularly in generating accurate impressions and handling nuanced clinical contexts, due to their training on radiology corpora [13, 14]. Furthermore, some institutions are piloting conversational AI in patient-facing radiology portals, where patients can ask questions about their imaging results and receive personalized, understandable

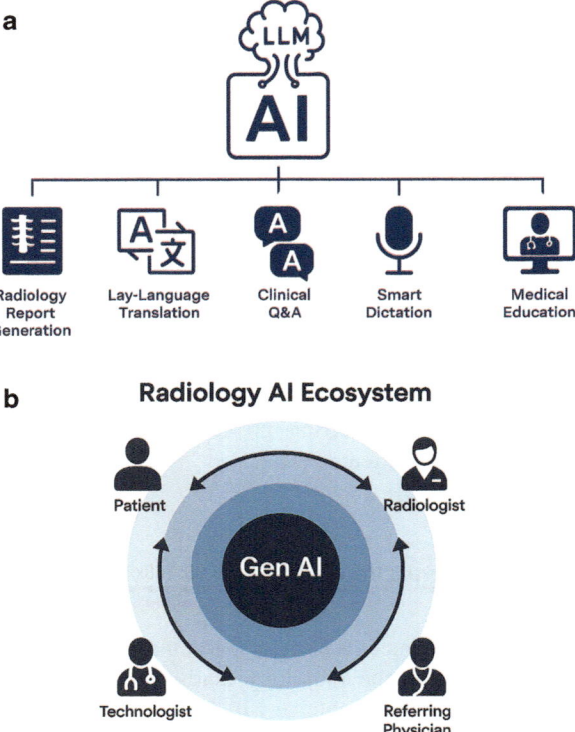

Fig. 47.2 Applications and ecosystem of generative AI in radiology. (**a**) Key use cases of large language models (LLMs) in radiology. (**b**) The GenAI ecosystem in radiology, highlighting its interactions with four primary stakeholders—radiologists, referring physicians, technologists, and patients—illustrating the multidirectional flow of information and support enabled by GenAI tools

explanations without requiring additional input from clinicians [10]. These advances have also extended to enhancing smart dictation, where AI not only transcribes but structures and edits reports in real time, aligning them with accepted standards like BI-RADS or PI-RADS [15].

Despite these promising applications, integration into routine workflows remains limited by reliability, bias, regulatory approval, and clinician oversight concerns. Nevertheless, the trajectory of generative AI in radiology is unmistakable—early research, pilot implementations, and user studies suggest that these models, with appropriate safeguards, will soon become indispensable tools for radiologists, educators, and patients alike [16–18].

Future of AI in Radiology

The trajectory of AI in radiology is rapidly moving toward multimodal models that combine imaging data with clinical context, including lab values, medical history, and genomics. These models allow for a richer, patient-specific analysis surpassing image-only systems' capabilities. For instance, transformer-based architectures integrating chest radiographs and clinical variables have demonstrated improved diagnostic accuracy and triage utility over traditional tools [19]. This evolution enables radiologists to shift from visual interpretation to comprehensive, context-aware decision-making.

Simultaneously, LLMs are enabling the rise of AI agents that can automate tasks like follow-up scheduling, radiology report generation, and personalized patient communication. LLMs could potentially be embedded within clinical workflows to improve efficiency without replacing human oversight—transforming radiologist-AI interaction into a true partnership [20]. These agents assist with structured reporting and lay-language translation and serve as real-time educational tools, supporting trainees with interactive guidance during case review.

Radiologists will increasingly function as "supervisors" of AI ecosystems—validating multimodal outputs, contextualizing AI-driven insights, and ensuring responsible use. While none of today's tools are fully autonomous, growing complexity and capability demand strong institutional governance and thoughtful integration. Emphasizing the importance of ethical oversight, technical infrastructure, and inclusive design can mitigate bias and promote equity in the deployment of LLMs across health systems [21]. With careful stewardship, radiologists are well positioned to lead this transformation.

For now, the technology has been integrated into the clinical workflow in very limited capacities, but it matures and evolves, more proposed use cases may become a reality. And none of the AI tools in radiology is currently fully autonomous; this will likely change in the future. Nevertheless, it is our responsibility as physicians and experts in this clinical specialty to maintain oversight of this new technology and ensure that it is used safely and appropriately for our patients.

References

1. Russakovsky O, Deng J, Su H, et al. ImageNet large scale visual recognition challenge. Int J Comput Vis. 2015;115:211–52.
2. Tadavarthi Y, Makeeva V, Wagstaff W, Zhan H, Podlasek A, Bhatia N, Heilbrun M, Krupinski E, Safdar N, Banerjee I, Gichoya J, Trivedi H. Overview of noninterpretive artificial intelligence models for safety, quality, workflow, and education applications in radiology practice. Radiol Artif Intell. 2022;4(2):e210114.
3. Moawad AW, et al. Artificial intelligence in diagnostic radiology: where do we stand, challenges, and opportunities. J Comput Assist Tomogr. 2022;46(1):78–90.
4. Harvey H, Topol E. More than meets the AI: refining image acquisition and resolution. Lancet Digit Health. 2020;396(10261):P1479.
5. Becker AS, Erinjeri JP, Chaim J, et al. Automatic forecasting of radiology examination volume trends for optimal resource planning and allocation. J Digit Imaging. 2022;35:1–8.
6. Daye D, Wiggins WF, Lungren MP, Alkasab T, et al. Implementation of clinical artificial intelligence in radiology: who decides and how? Radiology. 2022;305(3):555–63.
7. Elahi A, Cook T. Artificial intelligence governance and strategic planning: how we do it. J Am Coll Radiol. 2023;20:825.
8. Chen MM, Golding LP, Nicola GN. Who will pay for AI? Radiol Artif Intell. 2021;3(3):e210030. https://doi.org/10.1148/ryai.2021210030.
9. Lobig F, Subramanian D, Blankenburg M, et al. To pay or not to pay for artificial intelligence applications in radiology. NPJ Digit Med. 2023;6:117.
10. Zhang Z, et al. Patients' perceptions of using artificial intelligence (AI)-based technology to comprehend radiology imaging data. Health Informatics J. 2021;27(2):14604582211011215.
11. Tyson A, Pasquini G, Spencer A, Funk C. 60% of Americans would be uncomfortable with provider relying on AI in their own health care. Pew Research Center Report; 2023. Accessed 31 Aug 2023.
12. Andrews D. A patient's wish list for imaging artificial intelligence (and radiology). J Am Coll Radiol. 2023;20:868.
13. Jiang S, Xu Y, Lu X. ChatGPT in radiology: evaluating proficiencies, addressing shortcomings, and proposing integrative approaches for the future. Radiology. 2023;308:1.
14. Zeng W et al. Radiology-GPT: a domain-specific large language model for radiology; 2023. arXiv preprint arXiv:2306.08666.
15. Kunz WG, et al. Structured reporting in radiology: a model to enhance accuracy, efficiency, and quality. Eur Radiol. 2021;31(4):2140–9.
16. Ranschaert ER, Morozov S, Algra PR. Artificial intelligence in medical imaging: opportunities, applications and risks. Insights Imaging. 2019;10(1):1–19.
17. Johnson AEW, et al. Clinical question answering using large language models in healthcare. Npj Digit Med. 2023;6(1):45.
18. Tripathi S, Patel J, Mutter L, Dorfner FJ, Bridge CP, Daye D. Large language models as an academic resource for radiologists stepping into artificial intelligence research. Curr Probl Diagn Radiol. 2024;
19. Huang SC, et al. Multimodal chest radiograph analysis with transformers incorporating patient data. Radiology. 2023;308(2):e230806.
20. Tripathi S, Sukumaran R, Cook TS. Efficient healthcare with large language models: optimizing clinical workflow and enhancing patient care. J Am Med Inform Assoc. 2024;31:1436.
21. Tripathi S, Mongeau K, Alkhulaifat D, Elahi A, Cook TS. Large language models in health systems: governance, challenges, and solutions. Acad Radiol. 2024;32:1189.

Chapter 48
Disability and Life Insurance

Andrew T. Colucci

Life Insurance

Introduction + Definition

Life insurance is a contract between an insurer and a policyholder in which the insurer guarantees payment of a death benefit to named beneficiaries upon the insured person's death. The policyholder pays a premium, either regularly (e.g., monthly) or as a lump sum; the death benefit is a specified amount.

Life insurance aims to provide financial support for the policyholder's loved ones in the event of their death, to help them maintain their standard of living, pay off debts, and cover expenses such as funeral costs.

There are two primary types of life insurance policies: term and whole life. Term life insurance covers a specified time (e.g., 20 years). On the other hand, full life insurance provides permanent coverage and may include a savings or investment component.

As a rule of thumb, radiologists and future radiologists need to consider purchasing life insurance early in their careers, ideally while still in residency training, to ensure they have the appropriate insurance coverage when needed.

A. T. Colucci (✉)
Department of Radiology, Norwalk Hospital, Norwalk, CT, USA
e-mail: andrew.colucci@nuvancehealth.org

© The Author(s), under exclusive license to Springer Nature
Switzerland AG 2025
J. Shames et al. (eds.), *A Radiologist's Path*,
https://doi.org/10.1007/978-3-031-86882-5_48

233

Importance of Life Insurance for the Radiologist

Generally, life insurance is a valuable tool that can provide financial security for working professionals and their families in the event of their unexpected death. The death benefit from a life insurance policy can help cover expenses such as mortgage payments, college tuition, and other living expenses. Life insurance helps cover any outstanding debts or business expenses that may be left behind. In this way, it provides peace of mind for the insured and their family, knowing they will be cared for financially during their death.

For radiologists and other physicians, life insurance can be essential for several reasons:

Firstly, as a radiologist, one likely has high student loan debt from their medical education and training. A life insurance policy can help pay off these loans in case of the radiologist's death, providing financial relief for the family.

Secondly, the practicing radiologist may have a family to support. The death benefit from a life insurance policy can provide financial security for their spouse and children in the event of their unexpected death. Additionally, if the radiologist is the primary breadwinner in the family, the death benefit can help maintain the family's living standard.

Thirdly, a radiologist may have an ownership stake in a small business, like a private practice or a partnership. In the event of the radiologist's death, the death benefit can help pay off any outstanding business debts or expenses that may be left behind. This can help ensure the continuity of the business and provide financial security for the radiologist's business partners or employees.

Applied Examples of Life Insurance Policies

To illustrate the application of a life insurance policy, let's consider a radiologist with a wife and two children. This radiologist has a $500,000 remaining balance on their home mortgage, and both children plan to attend college in the next few years. The radiologist also has $100,000 in remaining student loan debt and fixed costs such as two vehicle loans, home utilities such as electricity, propane/oil, internet services, etc. In the event of the radiologist's death, their wife would be responsible for paying off these debts and covering living expenses for herself and their two children.

In this scenario, a term life insurance policy with a death benefit of $3 million would provide financial security for the radiologist's family. The death benefit would be used to pay off the mortgage and student loan debt, leaving the spouse and children with significant money to cover current and future living expenses. Additionally, the death benefit would help finance the children's college education.

As another example, consider a radiologist who is a partner and owner of a private practice. The radiologist's death would be a personal loss for their family and a financial loss for their business partners. A life insurance policy with a death benefit of $3 million would help to provide financial security for the radiologist's family. Still, it could also help to pay off any outstanding business debts or expenses that may be left behind. This can help ensure the continuity of the business and provide financial security for the radiologist's business partners.

Purchasing Life Insurance Early

It is advised that a radiologist purchase life insurance early, ideally while still in residency training, for several reasons:

Lower Costs

Life insurance costs are typically based on age, health, and lifestyle. The younger and healthier a person is, the lower their life insurance premiums will be. By purchasing life insurance while still in residency training, a radiologist can lock in lower rates and potentially save money over the long term.

Medical History

A radiologist's medical history is often considered when determining their life insurance premium. By purchasing life insurance while still in residency training, a radiologist can take advantage of their (presumably) good health and avoid potential rate increases due to medical conditions that may develop later in life.

Increased Coverage

A radiologist's income and responsibilities may increase as they progress. Purchasing life insurance while still in residency training allows a radiologist to increase their coverage as their needs change without going through the underwriting process again, assuming the appropriate riders are in place.

Peace of Mind

A life insurance policy can provide peace of mind for radiologists and their families. It can help ensure that their loved ones will be taken care of financially in the event of an unexpected death, even while they're still in the early phases of their career.

How Much Life Insurance to Purchase?

Determining the amount of life insurance to purchase can be complex, as it depends on individual factors such as income, debt, and projected future expenses. Here are some general guidelines to help determine the appropriate amount of life insurance:

Income Replacement

One way to determine the amount of life insurance to purchase is to calculate the amount of income that would be needed to replace the payment of the person who would be insured. This can be done by estimating the person's future income and multiplying it by the years that revenue would be needed.

For example, if a pretax annual income of 200,000 is needed for 10 years, then a 2 M dollar death benefit would be appropriate. Of course, this example is a bit overly simplistic, as the benefit could also be invested and provide additional capital gains/dividends over the years, depending on various factors such as market performance, which investments are chosen, etc.

Debts and Expenses

Another slightly varied approach is to sum all debts and expenses that would need to be covered in the event of the insured person's death. This can include mortgage payments, car payments, credit card debt, fixed home expenses, future college tuition for children, etc.

Future Expenses

A third component to consider is the incurrence and projected increase in future expenses. End-of-life considerations such as funeral expenses, assisted living costs, estate taxes, etc. are included in this group. However, one must also consider inflation and rising prices, as many goods and services will often trend higher over time. As such, the available cost of living will increase over time, and the insured's death benefit needs to be high enough to compensate for this projected increase.

Consult with a Financial Advisor

It's also essential to consider your goals, risk tolerance, and current financial situation when determining the appropriate amount of life insurance. A financial advisor can help you identify your specific needs and provide guidance on how much coverage is right for you.

Typical Cost of Life Insurance

The cost of life insurance varies widely depending on factors such as age, gender, health, lifestyle, and the amount of coverage. Added elements such as inflation and market conditions also play a role. The following guidelines are appropriate at the time of this publication.

1. Term life insurance: The most common and affordable type is term life insurance. It generally offers coverage for a specific period (e.g., 10, 20, or 30 years), and the rates are usually fixed. The average cost of a 20-year term life insurance policy for a healthy 30-year-old male is about $20 to $30 per month for a $500,000 policy. For a female, it's often somewhat less expensive.
2. Whole life insurance: Whole life insurance provides coverage for the entirety of the insured person's life if the premiums are paid. Whole life insurance policies are generally more expensive than term life insurance policies, but they also offer an investment component that can accumulate cash value over time. The average cost of a whole life insurance policy for a healthy 30-year-old male is about $100 to $150 per month for a $500,000 policy.

Evaluating Life Insurance Policies

When evaluating a life insurance policy, there are several things to look out for to ensure you get the coverage you need at a fair price. It's important to carefully review any policy and understand all the terms and conditions before signing up for coverage:

1. Coverage amount: Make sure the coverage amount is appropriate for your needs. Choosing a coverage amount that will provide the necessary financial coverage for your beneficiaries in the event of your death is essential.
2. Policy terms: Review the life insurance policy terms carefully to understand the coverage period, any exclusions, and all listed policy limitations. Make sure you know how the policy works and that it meets the needs of your and your family's financial situation.
3. Premiums: Compare the premium costs of different policies to ensure you get a fair price. Remember that the cheapest policy may only sometimes be the best option, although it often can be when it comes to level-term life insurance.
4. Policy renewal: Check if the policy has a guaranteed renewability option. This means that the procedure can be renewed at the end of the term without the need to pass a new medical examination.
5. Financial stability of the insurer: Research the insurance company's financial strength. The company should be financially stable and have a good reputation, which helps to ensure that they will be financially solvent and able to pay out claims in the future.

6. Options for additional coverage: Ask if any other coverage options are available, such as accidental death coverage, which pays out in case of death due to an accident.
7. Riders: Check if any riders are available for the policy, such as accidental death and dismemberment, long-term care, and critical illness coverage. Riders are additional pieces of add-on verbiage and policy components that are optional and may come with increased costs.

Life Insurance Riders: Several Common Examples

Accidental Death and Dismemberment (AD&D)

The AD&D rider provides additional coverage in case of death or dismemberment due to an accident. It pays out an additional benefit on top of the death benefit in the event of accidental death or loss of limb, sight, speech, or hearing.

Long-Term Care

This rider covers long-term care expenses such as nursing or in-home care. It allows the policyholder to use some of the death benefits to cover these expenses while they are still alive.

Critical Illness

A critical illness rider provides a lump-sum benefit if the policyholder is diagnosed with a critical illness such as cancer, heart attack, or stroke. The benefit can be used to pay for medical expenses or to supplement lost income.

Waiver of Premium

This rider waives the premium payments if the policyholder becomes disabled. This means the policy will remain in force without the need for further premium payments.

Children's Term

A children's term rider provides coverage for the policyholder's children at a reduced cost. It allows parents to purchase term insurance for their children, usually up to age 25, and the coverage will be automatically renewed each year.

Return of Premium

This rider allows the policyholder to receive a refund of all premiums paid if the policy is canceled before the end of the coverage period.

Spousal Rider

This rider allows the policyholder to purchase coverage for their spouse at a reduced cost.

It's important to note that not all riders are available with every policy, and some may be available at an additional cost.

Disability Insurance

Introduction + Definition

Disability insurance replaces income if the policyholder becomes disabled and cannot work. It is designed to replace a portion of the policyholder's income if they cannot work due to an injury or illness.

The policyholder pays a premium, either regularly or as a lump sum, and in return, the insurer will provide a specified benefit amount if the policyholder becomes disabled. The benefit amount is typically a percentage of the policyholder's income, and the length of the benefit payments may be limited or ongoing, depending on the specifics of the policy.

There are two main types of disability insurance policies: short term and long term. Short-term disability insurance provides benefits for a relatively short period, usually a few months. In contrast, long-term disability insurance provides benefits for a more extended period, typically until the policyholder reaches retirement age. Some disability insurance policies are also occupation specific, which means they are tailored to the specific needs and risks of certain professions, such as radiologists.

Whereas life insurance provides for your family and dependents in the event of your demise, disability insurance protects your income and financial future in case of an unexpected illness or injury that renders you unable to work.

Importance of Disability Insurance for the Radiologist

Disability insurance is essential for practicing radiologists because it provides income protection in case of an illness or injury that prevents them from working. A radiologist's income is often a significant portion of their overall wealth, and losing the ability to earn that income can have a substantial financial impact on them and their family.

Disability insurance can help replace a portion of a radiologist's income if they cannot work due to a covered disability. This can help them pay their bills, maintain their lifestyle, and provide for their family while they recover. Without disability insurance, a radiologist may rely on savings, investments, or government benefits to make ends meet, which can quickly be exhausted.

Additionally, disability insurance can cover new expenses such as rehabilitation costs or hiring in-home care. It also allows the radiologist to focus on recovery instead of worrying about finances.

Let's consider a radiologist who becomes disabled due to a back injury while weight training. They may no longer be able to perform the physical tasks required, such as operating imaging equipment or performing image-guided procedures. Without disability insurance, they may have to rely on savings or investments to make ends meet while they recover, which can quickly be exhausted.

In a study published in the Journal of the American College of Radiology in 2019, researchers found that radiologists had a higher risk of developing musculo-skeletal disorders (MSDs) such as back pain and carpal tunnel syndrome due to the physical demands of their job [1]. The study also found that MSDs can lead to disability and early retirement for radiologists. This highlights the importance of disability insurance for radiologists, as it can provide income protection in case of an illness or injury caused by their job.

Alternatively, a radiologist who becomes disabled due to a mental health condition such as major depression or anxiety may be unable to perform the cognitive tasks required, such as making diagnoses and interpreting imaging examinations. Disability insurance can provide income protection for them as well.

An article in Radiology Today in 2018 discussed the importance of disability insurance for radiologists, particularly those who are self-employed or own their practice [2]. The report noted that self-employed radiologists may not have access to group disability insurance through an employer and may need to purchase individual coverage. The authors also described that owning a practice can create additional financial responsibilities and obligations that must be met even if a radiologist becomes disabled.

It's important to note that many group disability insurance plans employers provide only cover a percentage of a radiologist's income, usually around 60%. There may need to be more to protect their total income and expenses. An individual disability insurance policy can provide additional coverage to supplement the group plan. Therefore, a radiologist may want to consider purchasing additional coverage, such as a personal disability insurance policy, beyond what the group policy provides [3].

Purchasing Disability Insurance Early

It can be necessary for a radiologist in residency training to purchase disability insurance early for several reasons. First, disability insurance premiums are also generally lower for younger and healthier individuals, so a policy is essential. In contrast, being in good health and at a younger age can result in significant savings over time. Additionally, purchasing a policy early in one's career can help ensure coverage is in place when needed most, such as in the event of an unexpected illness or injury that prevents the radiologist from paying off their student loan debt and establishing a nest egg [3, 4].

Furthermore, radiologists' careers often involve long hours of standing or sitting, repetitive motions, and radiation exposure—all of which may increase the risk of disability in the mid- to later career.

Finally, having appropriate disability insurance early provides peace of mind, allowing newly minted radiologists to concentrate on their work and training, knowing they have a financial safety net in case of an unexpected event.

How Much Disability Insurance Should You Purchase?

There are several factors to consider when determining the total amount of disability insurance to purchase:

1. Income: Primary factors are your current income and any relevant projected future increases. The goal is to have enough coverage to replace a significant portion of your income in case of a disability. A good rule of thumb is to aim for coverage that will replace 60–80% of your income.
2. Expenses: Consider your current and future expenses, such as mortgage or rent, car payments, insurance, and other bills. Make sure your disability benefit will be enough to cover these expenses in case of a disability.
3. Duration of the coverage: Think about how long you may need coverage in case of a disability. Some policies have a limited coverage period, while others will cover you for the duration of your disability.
4. Professional expenses: If you are self-employed, consider the additional costs of running your business, such as maintaining a practice, paying staff, etc.
5. Other resources: Consider any other resources you may have in case of a disability, such as savings, retirement funds, or a partner's income, and factor them into the coverage you need.

Typical Cost of Disability Insurance

The cost of disability insurance can vary depending on several factors, such as the amount of coverage, the length of the benefit period, the elimination period (the time before benefits are paid out), and the individual's occupation, age, and health.

On average, the cost of disability insurance can range from 1% to 3% of an individual's income. For example, a person earning $100,000 a year might pay $1000 to $3000 yearly for a policy. However, it's also important to note that if you purchase a policy while young and healthy, you'll likely pay less than if you are buying one later.

It's also worth noting that group disability insurance offered through an employer is typically less expensive than an individual policy. Some employers may provide coverage at no cost to the employee, while others may require the employee to pay a portion of the premium.

It's essential to remember that the cheapest policy may only sometimes be the best policy for your needs. It's important to compare policies and consider the features and coverage provided by each policy before deciding [5].

Evaluating Disability Insurance Policies

When evaluating a disability insurance policy, it's important to look at the definition of "disability" used in the policy. Some policies use an "own occupation" definition, which means that the policyholder is considered disabled if they cannot perform the specific duties of their occupation. Other policies use an "any occupation" definition, which means that the policyholder is considered disabled if they cannot perform the duties of any occupation for which they are reasonably qualified based on their education, training, or experience.

It is highly preferential for radiologists to select an "own occupation" disability insurance policy when possible. This means that if you cannot carry out the duties of a radiologist, specifically, you are considered disabled and eligible for the policy benefit. However, suppose you had instead opted for an "any occupation" policy. In that case, you may be denied the use if you cannot practice radiology due to an injury, so the insurance company could argue that you can still work a new and unrelated job (e.g., teaching medical students).

Beyond the definition of disability, several additional vital factors must be considered when evaluating a potential disability insurance policy [6]:

1. Benefit period: The policy should specify how long benefits will be paid out in case of a disability. Some guidelines have a limited benefit period, while others will cover you for the duration of your disability.
2. Elimination period: The elimination period is when you must be disabled before benefits are paid out. Look for a policy with a short elimination period to ensure you receive benefits sooner in case of a disability.

3. Benefit amount: The policy should provide enough coverage to replace a significant portion of your income in case of a disability. Check the benefit amount to ensure it covers your expenses, including any additional business costs if you're self-employed.
4. Renewability and portability: Look for a renewable and portable policy for life, meaning that you can keep the policy even if you change jobs.
5. Exclusions and limitations: Read the policy's exclusions and limitations carefully to understand what is not covered by the policy.

Disability Insurance Riders

Riders are additional options that can be added to a disability insurance policy to customize the coverage to meet the individual's specific needs. Several of the more common types of riders for disability insurance policies include the following:

1. Cost of living adjustment (COLA): This rider increases the benefit amount over time to keep pace with inflation.
2. Future increase option (FIO): This rider allows the policyholder to increase their coverage without providing additional evidence of insurability.
3. Noncancelable and guaranteed renewable: This rider guarantees that the insurance company will not cancel the policy as long as the premium is paid and that the policyholder can renew the policy regardless of changes in their health.
4. Residual or partial disability: This rider pays a percentage of the benefit amount if the policyholder can work but has a reduced income due to a disability.
5. Rehabilitation benefit: This rider pays for rehabilitation expenses, such as physical therapy, if the policyholder can return to work after a disability.
6. Waiver of premium: This rider waives the policy premium during the period of disability.
7. Return of premium: This rider allows the policyholder to receive a refund of all or a portion of the premiums paid if the policy is canceled or unused.
8. Catastrophic disability: This rider pays an additional benefit if the policyholder becomes disabled from a catastrophic event.

Summary + Key Points

Insurance plays a role in the overall financial strategy of emerging radiologists, acting as a hedge against catastrophe.

Level-term life insurance is a simple and relatively cheap product that will provide for your family and loved ones in the event of your early death, helping to cover costs, pay off debt, and reestablish their financial footing.

Own-occupation disability insurance supports you, your family, and your dependents in the event of your partial or total disability. While more expensive than life insurance, it will remove the burden of income production and allow you to focus on rehabilitation and recovery after an injury or disability.

For both life and disability insurance, purchasing an appropriate amount of coverage is recommended to meet the financial needs of your unique situation. For the above reasons, buying these products as early as possible is also advised, ideally while still in residency.

References

1. MD, et al. Musculoskeletal disorders among radiologists: prevalence and risk factors. J Am Coll Radiol. 2019;
2. S.B. The importance of disability insurance for radiologists. Radiol Today. 2018;
3. Findeiss L, et al. Issues most pressing to early-career interventional radiologists: results of a descriptive survey. Acad Radiol. 2022;
4. Gunderman RB, et al. Business education for radiology residents the value of full-time business educators. Acad Radiol. 2011;
5. Heilbrun ME, et al. Health issues and the practicing radiologist: defining concepts and developing recommendations for leave options and policies. JACR. 2013;
6. Keller EJ, et al. Disability in interventional radiology. Semin Interv Radiol. 2021;

Chapter 49
Conferences and Continuing Medical Education

Tessa S. Cook

Introduction

Continuing medical education is a critical part of the lifelong learning aspect of our profession. Radiologists in academia, private practice, government/military settings, and teleradiology are all responsible for continuing to maintain their knowledge and skills and learn about new advancements in their field. Continuing medical education (CME) credits are a formal documentation that radiologists are expected to maintain to demonstrate this commitment to lifelong learning. CME credits can be obtained by attending conferences, dedicated educational courses, or participating in the peer review process for scientific journals.

Conferences in Radiology

There are a large variety of conferences available to radiologists for the purposes of lifelong learning and continuing medical education. Some of these are offered by broad professional societies such as the Radiological Society of North America (RSNA), Association of Academic Radiology (AAR), and the American Roentgen Ray Society (ARRS). However, there are also a variety of clinical subspecialty conferences both within and outside radiology that offer CME and lifelong learning.

In addition, there are nonclinical subspecialty conferences, for example, those dedicated to imaging informatics or medical physics, that can also be relevant. There are even conferences devoted to professionalism that also offer CME. These

T. S. Cook (✉)
Department of Radiology, Perelman School of Medicine at the University of Pennsylvania, Philadelphia, PA, USA
e-mail: tessa.cook@pennmedicine.upenn.edu

© The Author(s), under exclusive license to Springer Nature Switzerland AG 2025
J. Shames et al. (eds.), *A Radiologist's Path*,
https://doi.org/10.1007/978-3-031-86882-5_49

include conferences related to physician wellness, professional development, career advancement, and mentorship of women and underrepresented minorities.

Radiologists generally have to be selective about the number of conferences they attend, as the clinical service has to remain sufficiently staffed while some radiologists are away at a meeting. Subspecialty radiologists may also have specific CME requirements for the field in which they practice that cannot be obtained at broader educational meetings and can only be satisfied by attending certain subspecialty meetings. Awareness of these requirements is important for remaining compliant with maintenance of certification.

Fundamentals of Continuing Medical Education (CME)

If you maintain licenses to practice medicine in more than one state, it is important to know each state's requirements for licensure and the schedule on which you have to earn CME to be eligible to renew each license. In addition, it is important to know what the American Board of Radiology (ABR) requires for maintenance of certification (MOC) [1]. Part 2 of the MOC requirements is currently titled Lifelong Learning and Self-Assessment and covers CME expectations. Detailed CME requirements from the ABR or individual states are not described here, as they may evolve with time and no longer be accurate by the time this chapter is published. Please refer to the relevant websites for the most detailed information on these requirements.

Similar guidance applies if you hold board certification in more than one subspecialty of radiology, e.g., both diagnostic and interventional radiology, diagnostic radiology and nuclear medicine, or Certificates of Added Qualifications (CAQs). Clinical informaticists certified by the American Board of Preventative Medicine also must earn special CME credits to maintain certification for that subspecialty.

Some radiologists have professional funds that they can use to cover the cost of conferences or CME courses that they attend as part of maintenance of certification. The funds may not cover all the credits required for a particular certification/licensure cycle; however, they will offset the cost to some degree.

CME for Conferences

CME credits are available for attending sessions at conferences and even for preparing presentations that are given at conferences. Individual conferences have different requirements for earning CME that may involve attendance in person versus online, CME offered only for sessions during the meeting even if enduring materials are available after the in-person time concludes, or CME that is available for many months after an in-person meeting ends.

It is important to check the specific guidelines provided by each conference to understand when and how to claim CME for sessions you attend. Some meetings may have session codes that need to be collected at the end of each session to claim credits. Most meetings will expect you to evaluate sessions for which you are claiming CME and provide input as to the quality of the speakers, the relevance of the content, the presence or absence of commercial bias, and any other relevant feedback.

Other Ways to Earn CME

In addition to attending or presenting at conferences, there are multiple alternative means by which one can earn CME.

Many peer-reviewed journals offer their reviewers CME credit for conducting a review that meets expected quality criteria [2]. This is because performing an effective peer review requires reviewing the existing medical literature and assessing the contributions of a new paper being considered for publication in light of work that has already been done. Most journals require you to request CME at the time that you submit your review.

Some conferences will also provide CME for reviewing abstracts or special exhibits submitted for consideration. For example, some conferences have an awards committee that reviews submitted presentations for eligibility for an award from the conference and offers the reviewers on the committee CME for their effort.

Research seminars, guest speakers, and grand rounds offered at academic medical centers also present radiologists with an option to earn CME. These are often regular sessions posted by specific departments throughout the academic year.

A variety of standalone CME courses also exist in radiology. Some of these are in-person meetings affiliated with large academic medical centers. Others are commercial products offered by standalone companies that compile lectures from subspecialty experts and present them as a subscription or standalone fee product that can be purchased and claimed for CME.

One benefit of membership in a professional society is often access to enduring content available online for the purposes of earning CME. This provides radiologists the opportunity to earn CME on a schedule that is preferable to them and from the comfort of the environment and location that they choose, without requiring them to travel if they do not wish to do so. The opportunity to earn credits for maintenance of certification may be time limited, so as to ensure that the educational material is not providing outdated information.

References

1. American Board of Radiology. Maintenance of certification for diagnostic radiology. https://www.theabr.org/diagnostic-radiology/maintenance-of-certification. Accessed 31 Aug 2023.
2. Kawczak S, Mustafa S. Manuscript review continuing medical education: a retrospective investigation of the learning outcomes from this peer reviewer benefit. BMJ Open. 2020;10(11):e039687. Published 2020 Nov 24. https://doi.org/10.1136/bmjopen-2020-039687.

Chapter 50
Maintenance of Certification and Becoming a Fellow of the ACR

Gilda Boroumand

Introduction

You've passed your certifying exam and are likely a few months into your first job as a radiologist. Congratulations! As a reward, the American Board of Radiology (ABR) has automatically enrolled you in the Maintenance of Certification (MOC) program. You'll notice that your ABR certificate states the date of your initial certification, accompanied by a statement that the "ongoing validity of this certificate is contingent upon meeting the requirements of Maintenance of Certification" [1]. It is in your best interest to stay vigilant about meeting MOC requirements throughout the year so that you're not left scrambling every March when the ABR requires that you attest to meeting MOC requirements.

The best resource on this topic is, of course, the ABR itself [2]. Here, I will break down the four components of MOC and provide some pointers on making this process less daunting. In the second section, I'll review how to gain fellowship to the ACR.

MOC Part 1: Professionalism and Professional Standing

This part is straightforward. You must maintain a valid, unrestricted medical license in at least one state (or Canada). If a licensing board takes any action against your license (probation, suspension, revocation, etc.), you must report this to the ABR within 60 days.

G. Boroumand (✉)
Department of Radiology, Norwalk Hospital, Norwalk, CT, USA
e-mail: gilda.boroumand@nuvancehealth.org

© The Author(s), under exclusive license to Springer Nature Switzerland AG 2025
J. Shames et al. (eds.), *A Radiologist's Path*,
https://doi.org/10.1007/978-3-031-86882-5_50

MOC Part 2: Lifelong Learning and Self-Assessment

This is where you need to hone your recordkeeping skills. The ABR requires 75 Category 1 CME credits every 3 years.

So how to obtain CME credits?

At most hospitals, you can receive CME credit for attendance at tumor boards, grand rounds, and other educational lectures. This is one of the easiest ways to keep up with CME. Most institutions record attendance electronically, and many will allow you to monitor your institutional CME credits online. If your institution does not provide you with easy online access to your CME credits, it is essential that you track your attendance yourself.

Journal articles, ACR Case in Point, and even non-radiology-specific online sources like Doximity are also ways to obtain CME credits. It would be best if you usually answered a few questions about the journal article or case to attain the credits.

National and regional radiology conferences are a great way to connect with colleagues and stay up to date with advances in the field while quickly racking up a large number (think 15–30) of CME credits. The RSNA, ARRS, and ACR annual conferences are top rated, and every radiology subspecialty organization has its annual conference. Some provide virtual options as well. The ACR also holds several monthly education courses virtually or at its education center in Virginia. Does combining a morning of learning with an afternoon of lounging on the beach or hitting the ski slopes sound more appealing? There are conferences for that, too. Keep these options in mind when negotiating your CME allowance. And don't forget that many conferences require you to claim credit for each lecture you attend—follow instructions and claim your credits before the cutoff date!

I suggest creating a spreadsheet with columns for CME sponsor (e.g., ARRS, RSNA, your hospital), course title, date, imaging modality, and number of credits to keep track of your CME. You'll want to keep PDF copies of your certificates if you're audited. Still, with a spreadsheet, you can easily track your progress in one place (and the documentation will come in handy for hospital credentialing and MQSA audits for those doing breast imaging). I also recommend CME Gateway (cmegateway.org), where you can aggregate all your CME from the major radiology organizations in one place. From there, you can run CME reports for any time frame. Individual organizations like ACR, ARRS, etc. will also provide you with a list of your CME activities on their websites, but it's convenient to have everything in one centralized site.

MOC Part 3: Assessment of Knowledge, Judgment, and Skills

You have two options for fulfilling the Part 3 requirement: participate continuously in the ABR's Online Longitudinal Assessment (OLA) or take a traditional exam every 5 years.

OLA requires some engagement for most of the year. First, you select the sub-specialties in which you want to be tested. Each week, you'll receive an email reminder to log in to ola.theabr.org and complete two multiple-choice questions. The questions expire after four weeks. You must answer 52 questions annually and may decline up to ten questions annually. Declined questions are not considered incorrect. However, if you answer fewer than 52, the unanswered questions will be regarded as "forfeited" and incorrect.

OLA is not graded on a curve. Each question is assigned a "passing standard" based on feedback from OLA participants who volunteer as question raters. Once you have answered at least 52 "scorable" questions, you will see your weekly cumulative score and weekly updates on your performance on the OLA dashboard. You will receive an annual performance evaluation (pass/fail) each January 1st after you have answered 200 scorable questions. The aggregate rating for your most recent 200 questions will determine if you are passing. If you need to raise your performance, you will have until the MOC annual review in March to answer more questions and keep your MOC Part 3 status as "Pass."

MOC Part 4: Improvement in Medical Practice

For Part 4, you must have completed at least one Practice Quality Improvement (PQI) project or activity in the previous 3 years. This can be an individual, group, or institutional multidisciplinary project or activity. The idea is to show engagement in efforts to improve system performance and patient outcomes. The ABR website lists many projects and activities that fulfill the requirement [3]. It's a good idea to check out the list of activities (which are too exhaustive to detail here) because they may be things you are already doing in your day-to-day work (participation in a certain number of tumor boards, for example, will qualify). You only need to attest to meeting this requirement. But you'll need to submit documentation if you're audited by the ABR.

Finally, you'll need to pay a MOC annual fee and attest to meeting all MOC requirements on the ABR website (https://myabr.theabr.org) every March. For the first 3 years after initial certification, you must only maintain a medical license and participate in OLA. Your first full annual review begins in your fourth year.

Becoming a Fellow of the ACR

You're not eligible for this yet if you're recently out of training, but it never hurts to know how to position yourself if you want to become an ACR fellow someday. Fellowship of the American College of Radiology is a prestigious honor awarded to about 15% of ACR members who demonstrate exceptional achievement in radiology. You must have a minimum of 10 years of post-training ACR membership and meet at least one of the following nomination criteria:

- Service to the ACR or organized radiology at national or local/chapter levels
- Outstanding teaching
- Significant scientific or clinical research

The application is on the ACR website. Each ACR chapter sets submission deadlines, which vary between April and June. You'll need to submit your CV, detailed documentation of your achievements in one or more of the nomination criteria domains, and 2–4 letters of endorsement from current ACR fellows (only one of whom can work in your practice). Applications are reviewed first by local chapters and then by the ACR Committee on Fellowship Credentials. Each candidate's credentials are measured against the nomination rubric (applicants are not competing against each other). Notification letters are sent in October, and awards are conferred at the convocation ceremony at the ACR Annual Meeting the following April. Check the ACR website (www.acr.org/facr) for the most up-to-date information.

References

1. Maintenance of Certification (MOC). The American Board of Radiology. https://www.theabr. org/wp-content/uploads/2019/01/MOC_Brochure_DR_IR-DR_RO_2019.pdf. Accessed 2 Feb 2023.
2. Maintenance of Certification for Diagnostic Radiology. The American Board of Radiology. https://www.theabr.org/diagnostic-radiology/maintenance-of-certification). Accessed 3 Feb 2023.
3. Participatory Activities. The American Board of Radiology. https://www.theabr.org/diagnostic-radiology/maintenance-of-certification/improvement-medical-practice/participatory-activities. Accessed 7 Feb 2023.

Chapter 51
Diversifying Your Career

Christopher Roth

Anything becomes increasingly mundane with repetition. While radiology is a diverse field in a number of ways, the practice of it is necessarily repetitive. In order to be efficient, radiologists tend to interpret the same type of imaging study repetitively in the course of a workday. In order to hone expertise, radiologists tend to focus on subspecialized subsections of radiology, restricting the practiced scope to a fairly narrow range of imaging studies. While every patient is different anatomically and medically and presents a diverse range of imaging findings, interpreting a narrow range of imaging studies in a dark room in relative isolation over decades might lose some appeal. Connecting this experience with the outside world of healthcare delivery provides value to both the outside world of healthcare delivery and the radiologist. Radiology is a niche field that is not well understood outside of the field, and, conversely, radiologists often do not appreciate the nuances of healthcare practice outside of radiology. Branching out as a radiologist pays dividends to the radiologist in terms of better understanding his or her role, and the value radiology adds to the healthcare system that otherwise does not understand the radiology perspective.

There are a number of ways to branch out and diversify your career beyond the practice of radiology. The academic environment offers tried and true ways to accomplish this through education and research. While these options are more challenging to pursue outside of academia, other pathways are more realistic outside of—and also viable in—an academic setting. Quality and safety are a ubiquitous need, and most departments feature a quality and safety infrastructure. Operational and business management of the practice are other critically important roles that benefit from radiologist engagement. Other important areas to consider include wellness and diversity, equity, and inclusion (DEI). Some of these roles are more

C. Roth (✉)
Jefferson Health & Thomas Jefferson University, Philadelphia, PA, USA
e-mail: Christopher.Roth@jefferson.edu

© The Author(s), under exclusive license to Springer Nature   253
Switzerland AG 2025
J. Shames et al. (eds.), *A Radiologist's Path*,
https://doi.org/10.1007/978-3-031-86882-5_51

clearly mapped out and provide a roadmap to acquiring the necessary skills and/or provide the requisite support; others are more nebulous.

While one stated reason for diversification is to stave off boredom and/or career stagnation, there are other reasons to consider this broadly. The obvious reason is to seek promotion, career advancement, and/or greater compensation. Other reasons include service to the department and institution and personal edification—learning more about the broader context in which radiology operates imbues the work with greater significance and renders it less rote. Just about any career advancement step involves assuming a leadership role with administrative responsibilities requiring at least some degree of expertise beyond clinical radiology. Some roles may require, or at least benefit from, formal education, such as quality and safety, research, and business management. All benefit from passion, interest, and relevant experience. No matter what path is chosen, at least some impact on daily routine is inevitable and should be acknowledged and accepted ahead of time. Committing to an educational program obviously incurs additional time and effort that has to be factored into the plan, and all roles beyond clinical practice add new tasks, time, and/or functions that distract from are added onto and can interfere with clinical practice. As such, the decision to embark on a formal educational or training program deserves, or at least likely benefits from, discussion with practice leadership because of the potential impact on flexibility, time, effort, etc. If nothing else, the advance notice will be appreciated and help to preserve and maintain better working relationships moving forward. Also, any perceived mutual benefit may lead to the possibility of sharing the cost of said program. Having said all this, pursuing degrees is addressed in an upcoming chapter, and the focus of this discussion is the broader topic of career diversification.

One of the greatest challenges to career diversification for physicians is the fact that it requires self-initiation and at least some degree of self-direction which is antithetical to traditional medical training which is heavily prescriptive (or at least used to be). Additionally, the career trajectory conforms to a conveyor belt in the sense that with acceptance to medical school and progressing along the educational and training path—albeit long and tedious—leads to a stable and at least fairly remunerative job. Diversifying a medical career is the opposite not only in the sense that it requires user definition and direction but also in that it lacks the clarity in terms of where it will lead. Some are imbued with certain interests and talents that naturally propagate them into career diversification, such as those with informatics skills that dovetail with the technology ubiquitous in radiology. Others may not have that built-in, opportunistic skill set or interest and still feel the draw or need to diversify. Part of the problem is that there are other skills that are very valuable outside of clinical practice that are often not recognized as skills. As Jocelyn D. Chertoff, MD, chair of the Department of Radiology at Dartmouth Hitchcock Medical Center, NH put it, "I learned that there are skills that I didn't consider to be skills, like running a meeting," Dr. Chertoff said. "I didn't know that was a skill.

I thought everybody could run a meeting."[1] This might be an oversimplification of scenario in medicine leading to career diversification opportunities, but the narrow focus on the scientific and medical aspects of the profession during the educational and training phases has left a monstrous deficiency of administrative, business, and other related skill sets required in complex organizations such as healthcare delivery systems.

Because physicians incubate in a classroom and then the institutionalized environment of hospitals under strict supervision generally with a steep hierarchy gradient, they tend to lack the experience others might gain during the earlier phase of their careers by interacting with others in the workplace in a more organic and less prescriptive fashion. Thereafter, the day-to-day routine of most radiologists is relatively more insulated from healthcare system operations and administration, playing out largely in isolated reading rooms. In order to catch up and understand the scope of possibilities, it is incumbent on radiologists to be as open as possible and take advantage of as many opportunities as possible—the exposure is the potential gateway to identifying compelling new roles or functions otherwise unknown. There is essentially no overlap between the learning and working environment in medical training and the clinical work of radiology on the one hand and the administrative oversight of healthcare systems or healthcare-adjacent entities. Rounding on patients as a cross-functional team might faintly resemble the kinds of meetings that occur outside of the clinical care realm, but with much greater freeform structure and organic process. In a sense, each individual patient discussion is analogous to a mini meeting where information is presented, there is some room for discussion (depending on the context, participants, culture, etc.), and action items are framed and assigned for completion.

Other "para-clinical" opportunities are also generally outside the confines of traditional medical education and training and routine clinical activities, such as participation on hospital committees (such as credentialing, privileging, ethics committees, etc.). For this reason, it is difficult to know whether such functions and activities are compelling and interesting, let alone whether the time investment is worthwhile. Therefore, an open-minded attitude is important to maximize opportunities for career diversification such as these. Exactly where such "para-clinical" opportunities might lead, if anywhere, is hard to predict, but they provide insight into what diversified work outside of radiology clinical work might look like on a day-to-day basis.

However, radiologists choose to diversify their careers; their "para-clinical" contributions to the field are critically important. The winds of change in healthcare are howling more than ever and the need to shepherd the profession along a rational and sustainable course is more important than ever. It is certainly better to lead oneself and colleagues than be led by others lacking understanding of the profession's needs, goals, challenges, and values. Radiologists in advocacy and government relation roles are able to articulate the needs of radiologists and the profession to

---

[1] https://www.rsna.org/news/2022/june/Unconventional-Career-Paths-Radiology

effectuate change. Radiologists in quality and safety leadership roles are able to quantify and measure the value provided by the profession and work with their team and others to elevate the quality of care provided. Radiologists in business management roles are able to understand the complex, dynamic relationship between the clinical practice and the economic realities. Radiologists in informatics roles are able to optimize IT operations and articulate the profession's needs to industry and healthcare leadership and partner with them to elevate the quality of IT products and services and thereby optimize and streamline the care and services we deliver. Radiologists in DEI roles work to increase diversity in the workplace and maximize diverse opinions and skills, promote inclusion and openness, and focus on reducing imaging-related healthcare inequities in society. These are just some examples of how diversification translates to value beyond the narrow confines of direct imaging care delivery; more familiar are the traditional examples of physician educator and researcher.

We all share a facility with science and medicine and specifically radiology, but we all possess a wide variety of additional attributes and skill sets that otherwise go untapped without career diversification.

Chapter 52
Leaving Your First Job and Finding Your Second One

Dana Amiraian

I grew up with parents who both had the same employer from before I was born until the day they retired. Times have changed, as most of my friends (doctors and nondoctors alike) have changed jobs at least once in our relatively short working lives. While I always envisioned myself remaining in the same position throughout my career, I am no different from my contemporaries—I am currently in my second job after completing my fellowship less than 5 years ago.

Straight from fellowship, I had what most would consider a dream job for a radiologist in private practice—Monday through Friday, 8 am to 5 pm: no nights, no evenings, no weekends, no holidays, and no call. The majority of my work was in my fellowship-trained subspecialty. The group was fair, and my colleagues were personable, business-savvy, competent radiologists. The practice was about an hour outside of my ideal geographic region, in a friendly community, close enough to visit family and utilize their occasional help for childcare. I had no reason to leave.

Then, the COVID pandemic started, and my toddler was no longer in daycare. I had another baby shortly after that. My husband and I had full-time careers and struggled to piece together childcare throughout the workweek. It became clear that we needed to be closer to family and adjust our work schedules to better balance the time demands of a young family while having fulfilling careers.

By sheer luck, I stumbled upon an open position at my former training institution—one predominantly focused on off-hours imaging, with evening shifts (not overnights) each week. The schedule would minimize our daytime childcare needs since my work schedule would only overlap my husband's for a few hours each week. This position also happened to be in the same city as extended family, who could then help out more regularly to fill the childcare gaps. I liked the institution

D. Amiraian (✉)
Department of Radiology, Mayo Clinic, Jacksonville, FL, USA
e-mail: amiraian.dana@mayo.edu

J. Shames et al. (eds.), *A Radiologist's Path*,
https://doi.org/10.1007/978-3-031-86882-5_52

and the radiologists, so pursuing this opportunity made sense. I was offered (and accepted) the job shortly after that.

Within days of accepting the new job, I spoke directly to the CEO and president of my private practice, letting them know I would be leaving. I was honest and open about why I was going and emphasized that I had a positive experience throughout my three and a half years working with the practice. I then called many of the partners to inform them personally before they heard through the grapevine or read about it in an email. Several of them thanked me for being professional in that regard. I fulfilled my remaining contractual time with the practice, conscientious through my last day. The course supported my decision and helped me understand my need to balance my family and career. I still keep in touch with multiple radiologists from the practice.

The decision to change jobs could not have worked out better for us. My schedule is atypical and a bit erratic, but it works for my family. I can do nearly all preschool drop-offs and pick-ups, and I have the freedom to volunteer for activities during the school day. I get to spend one-on-one quality time at home during the mornings with my toddler in these formative early years. The flexibility to schedule medical and dental appointments (and, yes, even an oil change) has been a boon for our family all while maintaining a full-time radiology career. An unexpected plus has been reconnecting with the world of academic medicine. I enjoy working with residents and fellows and collaborating with other radiologists and clinicians on complex cases. While this was an unexpected turn in my early radiology career, and I am grateful for my experiences in private practice, I am glad I took the chance and made the switch.

If you might be considering a change like mine, let me share some insights:

1. Stick it out at your first job for a while. That first year is a huge adjustment, especially those first few months, new practices, policies, people, workflow, imaging, dictation technology, and the angst of being alone for the first time. Any first job out of training will be intimidating. Give yourself grace and time to adjust. It may be time to look elsewhere if it is a toxic work environment or seems like a poor fit after a year.

2. If you are unhappy at your current job or it is not working for your life goals, assess your priorities. Identify the most important things to you as you search for your next job. Do you need to be in a specific geographic location? Do you prefer academia or private practice? Do you want to work remotely? Would you like to be fully subspecialized versus reading general cases? Do you want specific work responsibilities, such as procedures? Are you looking for a particular salary, vacation, or other benefits? Take these priorities into account when choosing your next job. As you rank your preferences, remember that life and your career change.

3. Consider that lifestyle and work-life balance mean different things to different people or at different life stages. For example, a Monday through Friday, 8 am to 5 pm, job may be ideal for having predictable and consistent free time during

evenings and weekends. Still, it would not be as flexible for daytime responsibilities.

4. Learn the lessons from your first job. You will undoubtedly grow as a radiologist while you navigate the early days of your first position straight out of training. Gain as much knowledge and first-hand experience as possible since you can apply this in your next job(s). In addition to the medical knowledge, learn what you like and dislike about your first job. Be honest about what you can or cannot live without (or tolerate) as you search for a new position. If you wish you had negotiated differently with your first job, use that experience to be better positioned to negotiate a contract for your next one.

5. Review your contract for your first job, particularly as it relates to noncompete agreements and tail coverage for malpractice insurance. Ensure the second job is outside the specified geographic area for the noncompete. Tail coverage is typically not cheap, so find out if you need to purchase your own tail coverage when leaving and then plan accordingly.

6. Secure your second job with certainty before giving notice to your first. The radiology job market is currently great but has ebbed and flowed historically. If you provide information with a new job solidly lined up, you avoid a potential gap in employment without income or other benefits, such as health insurance.

7. Leave your first practice on good terms as you move on. Give appropriate notice and complete any remaining work requirements outlined in your contract. During this time, maintain the same work ethic you brought to the practice on day one. They trained and relied on you during your tenure with them, so be respectful and professional for the practice and your patients. Plus, radiology is a relatively small community. A professional reputation is fragile, so do it right and remain on good terms.

8. Try to enjoy the process. Changing jobs is stressful, especially if you are trying to leave a toxic workplace, but try to view it as a chance to learn while embarking on a new chapter. You may remember a bit about yourself when you reflect on what motivated you to leave and what you hope will be better the second time. And though no job is perfect, you might end up exactly where you are meant to be!

Chapter 53
How to Advocate for Your Patients and Your Profession, the Ongoing Fight

Sharon L. D'Souza

"If you're not at the table, you're probably on the menu."

This is a principle I witnessed up close at an early age.

By having a physician parent, I grew up surrounded by physicians. Most social gatherings also included their physician friends, current colleagues, and former medical school classmates. As we all know, when you get a group of physicians together, there's inevitably some "shop talk" (often to the chagrin of just about everyone else). As a high school kid in the mid-1990s, I distinctly remember one such dinner where they all talked about this "crazy idea" being discussed in the state legislature. Optometrists wanted to perform eye surgery and were attempting to use the state legislature to expand their scope of practice.

As physicians, we are acutely aware of the vast differences in training and experience between optometrists and ophthalmologists. This is a significant oversimplification of the substantial training differences, however:

Ophthalmologists: 4-year undergraduate degree, 4 years of medical school, 3–4 years of residency, possibly 1–2 years of fellowship, oral and written board examinations.

Optometrists: 4 years of undergraduate degree, 4 years of optometry school. *note: does not include medical school*.

While I'm sure some defense was mustered in response to this legislation, I remember the prevailing sentiment at that dinner party is, "Of COURSE something like this won't pass; how could ANYONE think that this is in any way safe or appropriate? Allowing someone who has never been to medical school, someone without our extensive medical training, to perform procedures on the EYE? It will never pass." No one seemed especially concerned about this potentially dangerous

S. L. D'Souza (✉)
Tulsa Radiology Associates, Tulsa, OK, USA

J. Shames et al. (eds.), *A Radiologist's Path*,
https://doi.org/10.1007/978-3-031-86882-5_53

situation, fully expecting common sense, and the many legitimate concerns regarding patient safety to prevail.

Well, in 1998, the Oklahoma state legislature passed a law permitting optometrists to perform laser surgery procedures [1–3]. But wait, there's more! This bill also granted the Oklahoma Board of Examiners in Optometry the sole authority to decide what precisely constitutes the practice of optometry [2].

Subsequently, in 2004, in response to an opinion issued by the Oklahoma attorney general, lawmakers passed legislation that effectively removed traditional oversight bodies such as the governor, attorney general, and state medical board and their ability to regulate the practice of optometry [1, 2, 4, 5]. We can all guess what happened next. With their newly legislated authority and complete lack of oversight, the Oklahoma Board of Optometry passed a rule further expanding optometrists' scope of practice to perform surgical procedures on the eye [1, 2].

This was the first time I witnessed a group of people successfully circumventing the long-established, intensely rigorous pathway of medical school and residency, essentially legislating the practice of medicine by nonphysician practitioners (NPPs) despite the objection of multiple regulatory bodies put in place to protect patients.

Unfortunately, this was only the first of many such experiences. Once you start paying attention and your eyes have been opened to what is happening all around us, it is impossible to ignore.

On a positive note? This experience vividly demonstrated to me the importance of physician involvement and engagement in the creation of public policy as well as the importance of advocacy. I can't help but wonder what if legislators had been routinely hearing from physicians in the time leading up to this legislation? What if there had been such a public outcry at the blatant stripping of safety measures, holding legislators accountable, and putting their reelection up for debate that they could not afford to allow such legislation to pass?

I suppose this is what you call a "core memory." As a direct result of this experience, I have always taken the time and made an effort to remain actively involved in my county, state, and national medical/specialty societies.

"If you want to go fast, go alone. If you want to go far, go together."

Organized medicine can be a potent tool to amplify the voice of individual physicians. I have often become aware of pertinent legislation via my involvement with these organizations and my relationship with lobbyists. I have subsequently been able to raise the alarm and help rally physician efforts. Additionally, multiple physician grassroots efforts have played a crucial role in protecting patients and promoting physician-led care—Physicians for Patient Protection, Practicing Physicians of America, and Physicians Working Together.

Fast forward to another year, another state.

In August of 2017, in Washington, HB 1771 sought to create a "new health profession," Doctor of Medical Science, essentially allowing for physician assistants' unsupervised practice of medicine. Four physicians and I traveled to Olympia, WA, and gave strong testimony during the Department of Health Sunrise Hearing. As president of my county medical society, I testified and spoke on behalf of our board and our membership. We were joined in arms by the Washington State Medical

Association, the American Medical Association, the Washington Academy of Physician Assistants, the Association of Advanced Practice Psychiatric Nurses, and the Washington Association of Nurse Anesthetists. With the aid of social media and grassroots organizations like Physicians for Patient Protection, hundreds of letters and emails were written and phone calls made and were *directly quoted from* by committee members during the hearing.

In a testament to the immense power of advocacy and community organization—for the first time in the state's history—a bill was retracted immediately following this hearing, even before the sunrise review could be officially completed.

That same year in the neighboring state of Oregon, then Governor Kate Brown vetoed a psychologist-prescribing bill that crossed her desk, one which would have made Oregon the sixth state to allow psychologists to prescribe psychotropic medication. She correctly stated in a written statement: "There remains a lack of evidence that psychologist prescribing will improve access or quality of care. While prescription drugs may be appropriate mental health treatment for some patients, there are also significant health risks with some drug therapies [6, 7]." As a *direct result* of phone calls, emails, and letters from organized physicians spurred into action, she rejected an entirely inappropriate request to grant physician privileges to NPPs.

Some will tell you "this battle is already lost," that "the horse is out of the barn," and spending any effort to stem the tide of NPPs practicing MEDICINE and putting patients at risk is simply futile.

I'm afraid I have to disagree with this sentiment. This sense of hopelessness, helplessness, and push for complacency is not only out of touch and misinformed but also inherently dangerous—for us, our profession, and especially our unsuspecting patients. The path to adverse outcomes is often not paved with malice but indifference. All it takes is apathy, people looking the other way, and merely accepting a supposed inevitable result.

Physicians are patient advocates. We already advocate for our patients in big and small ways daily. Every time we encourage them to improve their health, for example, stop smoking or get their annual mammogram. How many physicians are in Congress? How many legislators genuinely understand the intricacies of what we do and what we struggle with daily? Unfortunately, they still need to pass laws that profoundly impact the practice of medicine. We need to be involved in making these decisions. Never forget that we are the medical experts. We need to take leadership. We must do the work. If we don't? It is simply not going to happen.

I encourage you to step out of your reading room. Please pay close attention to what is happening in our environment and keep one of your (expertly trained!) eyes on the horizon.

Do you remember your medical school application essay? Mine started with a quote from a 1990s movie, "French Kiss"—"I love the sea. So beautiful, so mysterious…so full of fish." I poured over it for months, trying to make it "perfect" and aptly convey my intense desire to become a physician. I still remember my "why," I bet yours is eerily similar because there's only one core reason someone would spend over a decade—a challenging decade—honing their craft. It's because you care. You care deeply about your patients and want to help them to the best of your ability. At its core, being a physician is about living a life of service to others. We chose to become the healers, the helpers, and the caregivers. Therefore, we are responsible for taking care of each other and our patients. I argue that responsibility is not confined to the reading room but extends far beyond.

Advocacy is simply an extension of this principle. Caring for someone means fighting for them. While this may at times seem like a daunting task, always remember—that ordinary people can do extraordinary things. And when we work together and focus our efforts? We can move mountains.

Worried you don't have time to spare? Leadership and advocacy come in many flavors—so grab a spoon and dig in! In less than an hour, you could, for example, meet with your institution's leadership or attend a webinar on your topic of interest. In 30 min, while waiting for your pizza order, you could write an email to politicians, or your hospital administration, write an opinion piece or letter to the editor, research, and consider supporting other physicians running for office. Paying dues and joining an organization or posting on social media takes less than 15 min. In 5 min, you could call a politician, donate money, or advocate for another physician. These time, money, and effort donations can have a lasting impact.

In the words of Madeline Albright, "I'm an optimist who worries a lot." We have every reason to worry; look to our emergency medicine, anesthesia, and dermatology colleagues and the ever-expanding NPPs' scope of practice. It would be the height of hubris to assume the same will not happen in radiology unless we take action. Additionally, there are compounding pressures from the administration, private equity, insurance companies, etc. Many external forces that rudely insert themselves between us and our patients are impacting our ability to practice medicine.

We will all be patients one day. If we don't try to right the ship, who will? Who will care for you and your loved ones when you are sick and vulnerable? While it may seem like the setbacks are many (and they are), do not let this decrease your resolve. Never stop using your voice to advocate for the good of your patients and your profession. One step forward at a time is enough; you will see progress in hindsight. And tomorrow? Well, tomorrow is a bright new day.

References

1. American Medical Association. AMA scope of practice data series: optometrists. Chicago: American Medical Association; 2010.
2. Hazel WA Jr. Oklahoma's optometrists encroach on surgical rights of ophthalmologists; place politics above patient safety. Arch Ophthalmol. 2005;123(4):559–60.
3. Oklahoma SB 1192, 46th Leg, 2nd Sess (OK 1998).
4. Scott RL. Health law perspectives: optometrists seek to expand the scope of practice privileges. University of Houston Health Law Policy & Institute. http://www.law.uh.edu/healthlaw/perspectives/RSShouldOptometristsPerformLaserSurgery.pdf. Accessed 10 Sept 2010.
5. Okla Stat Ann tit 59, sec 581(A).

6. Mapes J. Oregon public broadcasting. Oregon Governor to Veto 2 Bills, Plus Projects Sought By GOP Legislator – OPB. 8 Aug 2017.
7. Moran M. American Psychiatry Association. Oregon Governor Vetoes Psychologist Prescribing Bill | Psychiatric News (psychiatryonline.org). Published Online:12 Sep 2017 https://doi.org/10.1176/appi.pn.2017.9b3

Part V
Maintaining Your Health

Chapter 54
Maintaining Personal Health and Family Life

Ripple S. Patel

After a decade devoted to becoming a physician—amid school/training and making time for family/friends—we often forget to take care of the most crucial part, ourselves. Things will slowly fall into place once you start taking care of yourself. It can be a simple wellness routine involving enough sleep, eating healthy, and finding daily time for physical activity. If you can find an extracurricular activity that brings you joy outside of work and family, that is icing on the cake! Achieving happiness and success starts from within; it's an inside job.

With a clear mindset, you can better define your goals and purpose at any given moment. This will shift your priorities into focus. The focus may change occasionally, especially as you go through the life cycle and life transitions such as marriage, childbirth, sickness/death of a loved one, etc. Taking the appropriate time to reevaluate and reset your work and life goals is essential in finding the right work-life balance at that moment.

One of the biggest factors influencing your personal health and happiness with family life is job satisfaction. Finding the right job is like finding the right piece of the puzzle. If it's the wrong one, it will not fit no matter how hard you try. Ask yourselves what it is that strives you to grow professionally and find joy in your workplace. If the job description fits your needs perfectly but does not allow much time outside of work to enjoy, that may eventually lead to stress and burnout. The collegiality and support among your colleagues also play a huge role in having job satisfaction. Research in the field of work-life balance describes the spillover theory stating how a person's feelings, attitudes, skills, and behavior in one realm (work or personal/family life) can impact the other and vice versa. Spillover can have both positive and negative effects, and therefore it is important to find the right balance [1].

R. S. Patel (✉)
Department of Radiology, Thomas Jefferson University Hospital, Philadelphia, PA, USA
e-mail: ripple.patel@jefferson.edu

I personally do not believe that there is such a thing as a perfect balance. The major focus may shift from time to time depending on the situation. Your family life may also consist of many moving variables that are not under your control—such as your partner's job, children's activities/school, sickness, or taking care of an elderly parent. The key is to remember what your purpose is, and your priorities can be adjusted and shifted based upon the situation in order to maintain equilibrium with your personal health, family, and work.

I'll leave you with some pearls of wisdom that have helped me along the way and hopefully can do the same for you:

- Ask for help when needed, and take advantage of any help.
- Learn to say no to what no longer serves you.
- Life is too short to spend time with the wrong people and stay in a job that drains you.
- Don't wait for tomorrow—do what you can now.
- Don't take everything too seriously. Things have a way of working themselves out.
- Focus on your happiness in the present moment because nothing in life is guaranteed.
- Put yourself first—self-care is not selfish.

Prioritizing this last one has helped me the most. As a full-time working mom with young children trying to balance it all, this last one has taken me the longest to realize. This realization alone has become integral to maintaining personal health, happiness in my family life, and job satisfaction. Many of you may have heard the quote by Eleanor Brown, "You cannot serve from an empty vessel." Only once I find my own balance can I nourish my surroundings and hope to see them grow.

This may differ for each individual, but hopefully, it gets you thinking about what is essential. What brings you happiness? Let's start there as the first step towards maintaining your personal health and family life as you begin your journey after residency.

Reference

1. Bell AS, Rajendran D, Theiler S. Job stress, wellbeing, work-life balance and work-life conflict among Australian academics. Australia;2012. p. 25–26.

Chapter 55
How to Deal with Stress and Burnout

Chhavi Kaushik

Introduction

Stress is the physical and mental reaction to everyday challenges; every human being experiences varying degrees at some point. On the one hand, it is a normal reaction of the mind and body to external threats; it can become problematic if there is a constant state of physical and mental tension without any periods of relief in between. Burnout is a worldwide health problem that healthcare workers are not immune to. The latest definition, in WHO's International Classification of Diseases (ICD-11), says: "Burn-out is a syndrome conceptualized as resulting from chronic workplace stress that has not been successfully managed." It is characterized by energy depletion or exhaustion, increased mental distance from one's job, negativism or cynicism related to one's career, and reduced professional efficacy. Burnout refers specifically to phenomena in the occupational context and should not be applied to describe experiences in other areas of life [1].

Stress and burnout are prevalent among physicians in training and professional work settings. More than half of US physicians report some degree of stress and burnout in recent times. Physician burnout has been shown to increase the risk of substance abuse and suicide among physicians. It also compromises healthcare standards by decreasing physician productivity and increasing healthcare costs [2]. The Maslach Burnout Inventory™ (MBI) measures burnout as defined by the World Health Organization (WHO) and the ICD-11. The Maslach Burnout Inventory (MBI) assesses the level of burnout by measuring among physicians, including radiologists, the following parameters:

1. Emotional exhaustion: feeling emotionally overextended and exhausted by work.

C. Kaushik (✉)
Department of Radiology, Thomas Jefferson University Hospital, Philadelphia, PA, USA
e-mail: Chhavi.Kaushik@jefferson.edu

© The Author(s), under exclusive license to Springer Nature Switzerland AG 2025
J. Shames et al. (eds.), *A Radiologist's Path*,
https://doi.org/10.1007/978-3-031-86882-5_55

2. Depersonalization: unfeeling and impersonal responses toward one's service, care, or treatment recipients.
3. Personal accomplishment: feelings of competence and achievement in one's work with patients.

The MBI Individual and Group reports include suggestions for easing burnout, and the combined reports with the "Areas of Work Life Survey" suggest changing aspects of the work environment that might contribute to burnout [3]. The Areas of Work Life survey assesses what in the work environment may contribute to burnout by measuring workload, the opportunity to make decisions, recognition at the workplace, relationship with colleagues and subordinates, fairness and justice at the workplace, and alignment between professional and personal values.

Contributing Factors

The recent increase in radiologist burnout has been reported due to increasing workload, increasing after-hour responsibilities, greater expectations to meet RVUs open (relative value units), meeting turnaround time targets, conflicting demands of academic, clinical, and administrative roles, and struggles with suboptimal staffing [4]. An increase in the need for after-hour radiology reads led to enhanced recruitment of night-shift radiologists, resulting in a higher risk of burnout in the past few years [5]. Radiologist burnout has been reported in academic and private settings due to many contributing factors. Private practice radiologists reported higher emotional exertion, depersonalization, and lack of recognition [6], whereas in academic settings, the radiologists felt pressure to publish, obtain external funding, and meet deadlines for promotion and responsibility to teach trainees, interfering with their clinical duties and leading to professional dissatisfaction [7]. Radiologists, in general, were reported at a higher risk for burnout when compared to most other specialty physicians. Social isolation at work has contributed to radiologists' frustration and burnout [8]. A recent Medscape survey documented that 47% of radiologists reported having symptoms of burnout. It has also been reported that 54–72% of diagnostic and interventional radiologists suffer from burnout during their professional careers.

Unfavorable working conditions, including prolonged sitting in darkened rooms while interpreting imaging studies, gives radiologist a sedentary and stationary routine during work hours. On an emotional scale, this can interfere with circadian rhythm and contribute to sleep and mood disorders [9]. Longer sitting hours also contribute to chronic musculoskeletal pain, including joint inflammation and low back pain [10]. Women physicians have been reported to have a higher degree of burnout than men due to disparity in compensation, lesser opportunities for promotion and advancement, sexual discrimination, and greater expectation of familial duties at home than their male counterparts [11]. Burnout and stress are shared human experiences, an indication to reexamine our professional and personal lives and make essential changes to help us bounce back [12].

Solutions to Burnout Problem: What Can We Do?

Dealing with radiology physician stress and burnout requires personal, departmental, and organizational intervention. Restoring work-life balance and deriving satisfaction in all spheres of life is essential for the physician to feel empowered and work productively.

Radiologist Level Interventions

Studies have shown that even for radiologists who exercise daily, prolonged sitting hours have adverse health effects and slow one's metabolism [13]. People with active jobs can burn out approximately 1000 calories more than sedentary workers. An important concept to understand for sedentary workers is nonexercise activity thermogenesis (NEAT), a significant aspect of daily caloric expenditure. This excludes adventure sports, routine exercises, and energy consumption during eating and sleeping. Adding erratic movement and stretching exercises during a radiologist's day-to-day work can stimulate metabolism. Intermittently standing during working hours, as most radiology workstations are usually equipped with this feature, is a minor change that can be implemented to counteract the sedentary workflow. Adding extra walks and steps during working hours is suitable for physical activity, improves focus, and relaxes the mind [14]. One cannot undermine the importance of drinking plenty of water during the workday; this helps control weight and improves metabolism.

Additional lifestyle changes such as monitoring caloric intake, getting adequate undisturbed sleep (7–9 h), improving fiber intake, and eating early dinner at least 2 h before bedtime are simple steps toward positively impacting physical health. Taking care of one emotional and social well-being and incorporating healthy spiritual practices such as gratitude into daily life are effective stress-reducing strategies. Most institutions have employee health and wellness programs, which can be tailored to physicians' needs to ensure their physical and mental well-being. Radiologists should be encouraged to seek support from the peer group as well as counseling services. Taking proactive steps to spend time with friends and family helps counter work-related stress and improve work-life balance [15]. Grouped discussions during faculty meetings should be encouraged and serve a common purpose. Finding opportunities to volunteer and connect outside the workplace is equally important to improve quality of life.

Departmental and Organizational Interventions

Burnout has been acknowledged as a system-wide issue; departmental- and organizational-level interventions are much more effective in counteracting this problem. Modifications obtained in the work environment targeted toward enhancing positive social connections, being valued and supported, and being involved in workplace modifications to accommodate one's needs provide the most excellent chance of immediate impact [16]. The departmental leadership should frequently monitor working conditions, including worklist management, hours of work, accommodating flexibility, reducing interruption frequency, and mitigating skill mismatch to avoid any hindrance to radiologists' work engagements [17]. Open communication and transparency between an organization and staff are mutually beneficial to improve physician well-being.

Providing workflow autonomy by ensuring adequate staffing should be an organized-wide endeavor to avoid excessive pressure on radiologists to manage workflow. There should be clear policies on vacation benefits and coverage of significant life events such as childbirth, sickness, and bereavement [18]. Support should be provided for individuals deciding to convert from a full-time to a part-time position and vice versa. Proactive hiring of part-time and late-shift radiologists should always be considered to reduce the workload on the full-time staff [19]. Orientation at the time of joining and a continued mentor-mentee relationship between the new hire and the senior leadership is ideal to foster a sense of belongingness and improve professional satisfaction. This should be a constant effort to provide opportunities to become involved in professional activities of interest, such as clinical or basic research, involvement in professional ascites, actively participating in community artery programs, or undertaking administrative rules responsibilities [20].

Radiologists should be actively optimizing the electronic medical record system and PACS due to their workflow needs. A robust PACS and IT support should always be available to improve workflow quality and hospital-wide efficiency [21]. Continuous involvement in intradepartmental and intradepartmental conferences improves connections among radiologists and non-radiologist colleagues. Social events and holiday celebrations within the department and organization should provide opportunities to connect and destress. Meetings and get-togethers outside of work should also be encouraged [22]. Routine monitoring of physician well-being parameters with quantifiable measures is as important as patient satisfaction surveys. An enterprise-wide wellness committee is critical to assessing and evaluating per note at its earliest sign, making incorporating these wellness committees a popular feature among healthcare organizations. Regularly scheduled meetings at a generic level to improve the work-life balance of radiologists and a constant feedback mechanism is an important strategy to minimize the harmful effects of burnout for the physician and the organization [23]. Organizational leadership should always focus on implementing new techniques to impact radiologists' well-being positively.

Conclusion

Burnout is a real problem in radiology; an empathy toward the unique challenges a radiologist faces will aid in achieving insight and greater awareness toward achieving physician wellness, which will prevent and lessen the negative impact of stress and burnout. It is the moral duty of a leader and an organization to ensure that optimum steps are taken to address this global phenomenon. Times have come where this has become necessary for ensuring radiologists' job satisfaction, providing the best healthcare delivery, and obtaining the best healthcare for our patients.

References

1. Woo T, Ho R, Tang A, Tam W. Global prevalence of burnout symptoms among nurses: a systematic review and meta-analysis. J Psychiatr Res. 2020 Apr;123:9–20.
2. Chetlen AL, Chan TL, Ballard DH, Frigini LA, Hildebrand A, Kim S, Brian JM, Krupinski EA, Ganeshan D. Addressing burnout in radiologists. Acad Radiol. 2019 Apr;26(4):526–33.
3. Maslach C, Schaufeli WB, Leiter MP. Job burnout. Annu Rev Psychol. 2001;52:397–422.
4. Graham J, Ramirez AJ, Field S, Richards MA. Job stress and satisfaction among clinical radiologists. Clin Radiol. 2000;55(3):182–5.
5. Hanna TN, Shekhani H, Lamoureux C, et al. Emergency radiology practice patterns: shifts, schedules, and job satisfaction. J Am Coll Radiol. 2017;14(3):345–52.
6. Chew FS, Mulcahy MJ, Porrino JA, Mulcahy H, Relyea-Chew A. Prevalence of burnout among musculoskeletal radiologists. Skeletal Radiol. 2017;46(4):497–506.
7. Kelly AM, Cronin P, Dunnick NR. Junior faculty satisfaction in a large academic radiology department. Acad Radiol. 2007;14(4):445–54.
8. Spieler B, Baum N. Burnout: a mindful framework for the radiologist. Curr Probl Diagn Radiol. 2022 Mar–Apr;51(2):155–61.
9. Bender CE, Parikh JR, Arleo EK, Bluth E. The radiologist and depression. J Am Coll Radiol. 2016;13(7):863–7.
10. Daneshmandi H, Choobineh A, Ghaem H, Karimi M. Adverse effects of prolonged sitting behavior on the general health of office workers. J Lifestyle Med. 2017 Jul;7(2):69–75.
11. Stamarski CS, Son Hing LS. Gender inequalities in the workplace: the effects of organizational structures, processes, practices, and decision makers' sexism. Front Psychol. 2015 Sep 16;6:1400.
12. Canon CL, Chick JFB, DeQuesada I, Gunderman RB, Hoven N, Prosper AE. Physician burnout in radiology: perspectives from the field. AJR Am J Roentgenol. 2022 Feb;218(2):370–4.
13. Harolds JA, Parikh JR, Bluth EI, Dutton SC, Recht MP. Burnout of radiologists: frequency, risk factors, and remedies: a report of the ACR commission on human resources. J Am Coll Radiol. 2016;13(4):411–6.
14. Hoffmann JC, Mittal S, Hoffmann CH, Fadl A, Baadh A, Katz DS, Flug J. Combating the health risks of sedentary behavior in the contemporary radiology reading room. AJR Am J Roentgenol. 2016 Jun;206(6):1135–40.
15. Dyrbye LN, Sotile W, Boone S, et al. A survey of U.S. physicians and their partners regarding the impact of work-home conflict. J Gen Intern Med. 2014;29(1):155–61.
16. Simon AF, Holmes JH, Schwartz ES. Decreasing radiologist burnout through informatics-based solutions. Clin Imaging. 2020 Feb;59(2):167–71.
17. Bailey CR, Bailey AM, McKenney AS, Weiss CR. Understanding and appreciating burnout in radiologists. Radiographics. 2022 Sep–Oct;42(5):E137–9.

18. Bonner L. Radiologists are burning out. Diagnostic Imaging. 4 June 2015.
19. Bluth EI, Bansal S. The 2016 ACR Commission on human resources workforce survey. J Am Coll Radiol. 2016;13(10):1227–32.
20. Shanafelt TD, West CP, Sloan JA, et al. Career fit and burnout among academic faculty. Arch Intern Med. 2009;169(10):990–5.
21. Anderson M. The impact of university provided nurse electronic medical record training on health care organizations: an exploratory simulation approach. In: Driving quality in informatics: fulfilling the promise. 2015. Vol. 208, p. 1.
22. Cracknell ALA, Winfield A, Arkhipkina S, McDonagh E, Green A, Rooney M. Huddle up for safer healthcare: how frontline teams can work together to improve patient safety. Future Healthcare J. 2016;3(2):s31.
23. Snipes RL, Loughman T, Fleck RA. The effects of physicians' feelings of empowerment and service quality perceptions on hospital recommendations. Qual Manag J. 2010;17(4):51.

Chapter 56
When Is a Good Time to Have a Baby?

Anne Kathryn Misiura

When is a good time to have a baby?

Trick question. There is no "good" time.

I could fill an entire book on the timing of becoming a parent, but as you're here about how it pertains to a career in radiology, let me focus this wild topic down a bit.

I'll start by mentioning that my credentials consist of being a mom to a 3.5 year old I delivered during the first year of my first real attending job (and a 5 month old), whose favorite toy is the PowerMic on my home workstation. My first bit of advice is to have a backup PowerMic as a distraction. Remember this if you remember nothing else.

Assuming you're already in residency and have found yourself childless, you have a two options: having a kid in residency/fellowship or waiting until later. As of July 2022, the Accreditation Council for Graduate Medical Education (ACGME) requires programs to offer their trainees six weeks of paid medical, parental, and caregiver leave [1]. At least one week of allotted vacation time per year for all residents must be outside these six weeks. This additional clarification ensures that programs do not force you to use up all of your vacation time with this parental leave. This should not interfere with your graduation date. You can also have an additional unpaid 12 weeks of FMLA time off. This will interfere with your graduation date and with your board eligibility timing.

Most people will agree that 6 weeks is not enough time off, particularly if you're the gestating parent. But the thought of pushing back graduation by taking more time with FMLA (and thus dealing with off-cycle fellowship start and later board eligibility) sounds like a headache. This is enough reason for some to forgo having a child while in residency. But let me mention a few reasons you might choose to do so anyway:

A. K. Misiura (✉)
Department of Radiology, Thomas Jefferson University Hospital, Philadelphia, PA, USA
e-mail: anne.misiura@jefferson.edu

© The Author(s), under exclusive license to Springer Nature Switzerland AG 2025
J. Shames et al. (eds.), *A Radiologist's Path*,
https://doi.org/10.1007/978-3-031-86882-5_56

- You and your partner are not getting any younger. Females, in particular, in medicine, are at risk for higher infertility rates than the general population [2]. The older you are, the harder it may be to procreate.
- Your partner is at a point in their life/career where they are able and willing to be the primary caregiver.
- You may know you want 2.5 kids and want to do it asap.
- You have childcare help in the area—family, friends, or whomever.
- Daycare hours are amenable to you. Radiology residency isn't an 80-hour work week. Most of your rotations are during general business hours, so childcare pick up and drop off is easier for you than your anesthesiology or surgery resident pals.
- Programs will find coverage while you're out. Getting coverage might not be as easy for your practice as attending. But either way, it should never fall on you to find the coverage.
- Your family planning includes the need for reproductive assistance, which is a long process. Your insurance coverage while in residency covers some or all IVF/IUI/embryo freezing costs, etc. More than likely, it does not, in which case you may choose to wait until you're an attending and have a higher income level.

More reasons may be individual to you. But the point is, if you could make it work during residency, then make it work. Life is short.

Now, for the flip side, waiting until you're an attending can seem like the ideal choice for some. And maybe it's the *only* choice if you've been living apart from your partner during your training. You're not worrying about any future timeline disruption as no "graduation date" looms. There are potentially more opportunities to work from home or create more flexible hours and hybrid schedules, including working part-time so that you can be around more for the youngest years.

All the other points I mentioned supporting having a child during residency might apply when you're an attending instead. Maybe you've settled down for your first job close to family, so grandparents, aunts, and uncles are a phone call away for emergency childcare. You're more able to afford a nanny or au pair, so you have hands-on help to make your daily life less stressful.

If you need reproductive assistance, removing the worry of financial strain is a big draw to waiting until you're an attending. But again, I must mention that this process can be long, and there are no guarantees. Time is undoubtedly a critical variable that is not on your side.

Parenthood, and the path to becoming a parent, is not a one-size-fits-all experience. There is no good time to have a baby. So, do it when you want. You can make it work.

And don't forget that extra PowerMic.

References

1. ACGME Institutional Requirements [Internet]. [cited 2023 Feb 22]. https://www.acgme.org/globalassets/pfassets/programrequirements/800_institutionalrequirements2022.pdf
2. Stentz NC, Griffith KA, Perkins E, Jones RDC, Jagsi R. Fertility and childbearing among American female physicians. J Women's Health. 2016;25(10):1059–65.

Chapter 57
Developing and Maintaining Interests Outside of Medicine

Chhavi Kaushik

Introduction

Developing and maintaining interests outside of medicine is a great way to boost the quality of a physician's life, both inside and outside the work setting. With increasing responsibilities in the professional role with each transition and compartment of personal life, almost half of the radiologist physicians complain of burnout. Developing hobbies that enrich one's life is a way to gauge self-care and wellness in physicians. Physicians are human first, and it is important to identify individual needs and continue fostering interest guided by passion. Maintaining enjoyable hobbies not only releases stress but can also help with social networking, which is more pertinent to a radiologist given the routinely felt isolation at work. Spending free time on activities of interest is essential, which helps maintain balance, improves health, relieves stress, and allows self-expression. In this chapter, we will discuss some examples of fabulous hobbies for radiologists, leading to a healthier, happier, and more productive life [1].

Yoga, Meditation, and Mindfulness

Anxiety and stress can implode a radiologist's daily work due to endless documentation, answering multiple phone calls, and continuously making high stake decisions. Yoga, meditation, and mindfulness are retreats for the mind and body and have recently been incorporated as a part of physician wellness among organizations. Breath work during yoga entails bringing sense to the present moment,

C. Kaushik (✉)
Department of Radiology, Thomas Jefferson University Hospital, Philadelphia, PA, USA
e-mail: Chhavi.Kaushik@jefferson.edu

© The Author(s), under exclusive license to Springer Nature Switzerland AG 2025
J. Shames et al. (eds.), *A Radiologist's Path*,
https://doi.org/10.1007/978-3-031-86882-5_57

helping in increasing awareness, and relieving stress and anxiety. Yoga also improves symptoms in people with chronic pain, including low back pain [2]. Mindfulness and medications have a beneficial effect in lowering stress, counteracting burnout and depression, and positively impacting a person's life. Research has shown better moods, attentiveness, and overall improvement in the quality of life of healthcare professionals engaged in such practices [3].

Outdoor Activities, Including Cycling, Hiking, and Camping

Nature-based social activities are known to improve connectedness, strengthen the social structure, and help to alleviate the loneliness epidemic growing in the USA. Especially for radiologists, where a sedentary lifestyle comes with specific negative health effects, being actively involved on a routine basis in outdoor physical activities has positive physical and mental health benefits [4]. Studies have shown decreased blood pressure, lower stress levels, and improved immune functions in people who spent more time in physical activities engaging with nature. National and state parks adequate with biking trails, hiking routes with maps, and camping grounds have started to partner ring with healthcare professionals to promote outdoor on major related activities. This is a great time to connect with nature and have quality family time [5].

Reading and Writing

Reading as a hobby is "a pursuit outside one's regular occupation, especially for relaxation." Reading can expand horizons and be entertaining as there is always something new to enjoy. Reading can be done anytime, is inexpensive, and enhances knowledge. Reading is an all-inclusive hobby that requires no skill set and can be done as a family or social activity. People who read have better cognition, and recent research shows decreased incidence of dementia in later life [6, 7]. Writing is an excellent hobby with which one can explore one's creativity, and writing slows one down, instilling thoughtfulness. One can join reading and writing groups to share thoughts and ideas, join book clubs to develop this habit, and enhance social interactions.

Playing Musical instrument

Playing a musical instrument can be a way to find ease in complex life situations, grounding oneself in times of stress and anxiety, and be a healthy way to entertain. Apart from this, playing a musical instrument increases blood flow to the middle cerebral artery and improves cognitive abilities [7, 8]. Music relieves stress, lowers blood pressure, and helps combat insomnia. Music is a great way to connect with others and weave meaningful interpersonal relationships. Learning to play a musical instrument opens portals to lifelong enjoyment and learning. There is no wrong age to start learning a musical instrument, with so many online learning opportunities and apps which provide learning a musical instrument from the comfort of one's home. Harmonica is one of the easiest-to-learn musical instruments, others including guitar, ukulele, drums, and keyboards.

Financial Planning and Investment

One of the most remunerative hobbies a physician can have is doing financial planning and investments. A physician needs to save a portion of their incomes for investment purposes. Learning to invest as a physician, be it stock market or real estate, will require interest, time, and some degree of dedication. It's a wise choice of hobby for those who feel inclined, as it's both enjoyable and profitable. Some consider learning to manage their investments easier than learning medicine. One may initially consider hiring a financial advisor and then start learning the process. Some recent researchers have concluded that personal financial basics, estate planning, stock market investment, and retirement planning should be added to the medical school training curriculum. Physicians handling their financial investments consider this the best-paying hobby [9, 10].

Traveling

The Cambridge Dictionary definition of a hobby is "an activity someone does for pleasure when they are not working." Traveling can be a great hobby to enhance pleasure and take a break from mundane life. Traveling allows one to see places one has not seen and experience other cultures. Physicians can find creative ways to go off the traditional path and add travel adventures to their medical journey. There are always opportunities to attend medical conferences in different parts of the world. Increasing active travel has widely known health benefits and reduces the risks of obesity [11]. This is also a great way to meet new people and share interesting stories about each other's lives. Also, the component of unpredictability can add adventure to travel, and these help one rejuvenate and keep their spirit alive [11]. Travel can also be relaxing and distressing.

Artwork and Painting

Painting as a hobby enhances fine motor skills, boosts one's self-esteem, helps to relax the mind, and cultivates imagination. Few people find art as a form of meditation and disengagement from the world. Paintings have a rich culture and history and as a hobby act as a medium to connect with others. Art and painting help engage one's attention and improves self-esteem and social behavior. Art has been therapeutic in patients with dementia and mental health issues, including anxiety and depression [12].

Dancing

Dancing is one of the best ways to exercise the body and relax the mind, as it integrates movement and cognition [13, 14]. Dancing expresses joy; partner dance is one of the best forms of human-to-human connection. Dancing helps in emotional regulation and is a huge confidence booster. Dancing is one of the oldest and most popular forms of art.

Gardening

Gardening is an activity that is good for both mind and body. Planting and growing flowers and vegetables can benefit humanity and the environment in many ways. Spending time in the green zone has substantial mental and physical health benefits. It can be picked at any location and can be done around the year. One can derive pleasure from eating home-grown organic foods [15].

Playing Sports

Sports has always been a popular and enjoyable hobby with many physical and mental health benefits. Physical sports popularly played as hobbies include football, basketball, billiards, tennis, and golf. Mental sports include chess, solving crossword puzzles, and Sudoku. Sports genuinely help a person to learn about themselves. Strategizing and planning as a part of team sports helps keeps the mind sharp and opens windows to connect with others for a common goal [16].

Hobbies are a means to gain recreation, be a source of pleasure, and help pass free time. Physicians should have some hobbies, specifically in today's strenuous and demanding healthcare environment. Hobbies not only enlighten us but also provide essential vitality boost to progress in our professional life.

References

1. Ahmad A. Managing physician fatigue. Gastrointest Endosc Clin N Am. 2021 Oct;31(4):641–53.
2. Chou R, Deyo R, Friedly J, Skelly A, Hashimoto R, Weimer M, Fu R, Dana T, Kraegel P, Griffin J, Grusing S, Brodt ED. Nonpharmacologic therapies for low back pain: a systematic review for an American College of physicians clinical practice guideline. Ann Intern Med. 2017 Apr 4;166(7):493–505.
3. Chmielewski J, Łoś K, Łuczyński W. Mindfulness in healthcare professionals and medical education. Int J Occup Med Environ Health. 2021 Jan 7;34(1):1–14.
4. Leavell MA, Leiferman JA, Gascon M, Braddick F, Gonzalez JC, Litt JS. Nature-based social prescribing in urban settings to improve social connectedness and mental well-being: a review. Curr Environ Health Rep. 2019 Dec;6(4):297–308.
5. Mitten D, Overholt JR, Haynes FI, D'Amore CC, Ady JC. Hiking: a low-cost, accessible intervention to promote health benefits. Am J Lifestyle Med. 2016 Jul 9;12(4):302–10.
6. Kangassalo L, Spapé M, Ravaja N, Ruotsalo T. Information gain modulates brain activity evoked by reading. Sci Rep. 2020 May 6;10(1):7671.
7. Marshall R. Reading fiction: the benefits are numerous. Br J Gen Pract. 2020 Jan 30;70(691):79.
8. Kawasaki A, Hayashi N. Playing a musical instrument increases blood flow in the middle cerebral artery. PLoS One. 2022 Jun 8;17(6):e0269679.
9. Roberts WC. The importance of acquiring financial security for physicians. Am J Med. 2020 Dec;133(12):1403–5.
10. Doroghazi RM. Investing 101: how to achieve financial security. Am J Cardiol. 2019 Jul 15;124(2):312.
11. Saunders LE, Green JM, Petticrew MP, Steinbach R, Roberts H. What are the health benefits of active travel? A systematic review of trials and cohort studies. PLoS One. 2013 Aug 15;8(8):e69912.
12. Chancellor B, Duncan A, Chatterjee A. Art therapy for Alzheimer's disease and other dementias. J Alzheimers Dis. 2014;39(1):1–11.
13. Koch SC, Riege RFF, Tisborn K, Biondo J, Martin L, Beelmann A. Effects of dance movement therapy and dance on health-related psychological outcomes. A meta-analysis update. Front Psychol. 2019 Aug 20;10:1806.
14. Teixeira-Machado L, Arida RM, de Jesus MJ. Dance for neuroplasticity: a descriptive systematic review. Neurosci Biobehav Rev. 2019 Jan;96:232–40.
15. Ainamani HE, Gumisiriza N, Bamwerinde WM, Rukundo GZ. Gardening activity and its relationship to mental health: understudied and untapped in low-and middle-income countries. Prev Med Rep. 2022 Aug 8;29:101946.
16. Oja P, Titze S, Kokko S, Kujala UM, Heinonen A, Kelly P, Koski P, Foster C. Health benefits of different sport disciplines for adults: systematic review of observational and intervention studies with meta-analysis. Br J Sports Med. 2015 Apr;49(7):434–40.

Chapter 58
Life as a Radiologist from a Spouse's Perspective

Amit Patel and Ripple S. Patel

Shall we begin with the most common and often confusing question: What exactly does a Radiologist do? If you had asked me before dating and then marrying my Radiologist spouse, I would've said, "Ummm, look at X-rays, I think." After all these years, I've come to realize there's much more to it than that. However, it can still be a bit perplexing for those who aren't familiar with the field. The most common is the group of friends/family that call my spouse to ask about every physical ailment they have. I have colleagues and friends of my own who reach out and ask me to get my spouse's opinion on issues they are having. To draw a parallel, I work in the software industry and have yet to receive a call from anyone of relevance asking me about syntax errors they are having. I recently learned that my spouse would be privileged to work from home during specific periods. As someone who also works from home, this caused a constraint in both my Internet connection (those enormous Tomosynthesis file sizes) and the eviction notice from my office. The office, previously known as mine, has now been turned into a dark room that gets used infrequently for work and serves as a quaint retreat from people. This led me to a humorous conclusion on the work life of a Radiologist. You have worked so hard to end up in a dark solitary space that doubles as an escape from people! Jokingly, of course, there is a constant theme of dark and lonely here that must be addressed in another chapter.

As a spouse, I can't help but to realize there is another factor in our relationship, the kids. We have two incredible girls who absolutely adore my Radiologist spouse. So much so that every year since the school began, they've been asked to complete an "about me" bio for their teacher and classmates to help everyone get to know one

A. Patel
Spouse of a Radiologist, Moorestown, NJ, USA

R. S. Patel (✉)
Department of Radiology, Thomas Jefferson University Hospital, Philadelphia, PA, USA
e-mail: ripple.patel@jefferson.edu

© The Author(s), under exclusive license to Springer Nature Switzerland AG 2025
J. Shames et al. (eds.), *A Radiologist's Path*,
https://doi.org/10.1007/978-3-031-86882-5_58

another. Every year the question is posed, "What do you want to be when you grow up?" Their answer is always and without fail, a Radiologist.

Like seriously, what does a preschooler even know about Radiology?

This profession has engulfed my kids so that nobody even cares to ask what I do! Now, you'd assume this is a concern for a spouse; ironically, I love it. As mentioned, I find Radiology a fantastic field - one that no one just stumbles into. You have to be intelligent, have a strong work-ethic, make life-changing diagnoses, be empathetic, and for some reason I still don't fully understand—be good at physics. If our kids can have these attributes, then as both a parent and a spouse, I wouldn't trade my spouse's profession for anything.

We know a lot of professionals, both in the medical field and beyond, and as a spouse of a Radiologist, comparatively, it's a nice change of pace to see the job day in and day out bring my spouse joy. Let's face it, your job as a Radiologist deals with people's lives and well-being; you aren't writing code or changing the colors on a spreadsheet—this job truly matters, and my spouse handles it with grace. Also, working hours usually range from 8 to 5, despite the force out of the dark into the light; you cannot beat that for a physician.

To all the Radiologist spouses out there, give your spouse the acknowledgment they deserve from time to time - or whenever they force you to write a few words for some book you've never heard of, whichever comes first. The strange scenarios you face are all worth it when you end up on a beach somewhere relaxing while your spouse is attending Radiology conference sessions.

Chapter 59
Balancing Your Career with Family

Dana Amiraian

I always knew I would be a doctor, and I always knew I would be a wife and mother. I have since learned from experience that balancing a radiology career and a family is complex, evolving, and attainable.

I had my first child in the second half of my fellowship year. Fortunately, I had a flexible and understanding training program, which allowed me to coordinate vacation and research time to maximize time at home with my new baby while still being productive. I used my last few months of fellowship to hone my subspecialty radiology skills and become more comfortable working as a full-time radiologist with a baby at home. This eased my transition to private practice because I was used to leaving my child with another caregiver while I went to work.

Our daughter attended full-time daycare while my husband and I worked. She was well cared for and could learn and socialize through engaging in daily activities. She also caught countless viruses and was homesick, seemingly as often as she attended daycare. Thankfully my husband's job was relatively flexible, and we had family willing to help with childcare when our daughter could not participate in daycare.

Of course, things became more complicated when the COVID pandemic began, as our daughter was no longer in daycare. I had our second daughter early in the pandemic, so I took advantage of the unexpected societal upheaval and extended my maternity leave to spend more dedicated time at home with my young children. By the end of my maternity leave, I felt ready to return to my full-time career. Due to the pandemic, we arranged for extended family to care for our children upon my return to work.

My private practice schedule was 8 am to 5 pm, Monday through Friday. Despite the seemingly perfect standard work schedule, I had limited flexibility to take time

D. Amiraian (✉)
Department of Radiology, Mayo Clinic, Jacksonville, FL, USA
e-mail: amiraian.dana@mayo.edu

J. Shames et al. (eds.), *A Radiologist's Path*,
https://doi.org/10.1007/978-3-031-86882-5_59

off for a sick child or a pediatrician appointment at the last minute. I also missed most of my children's waking hours, which did not work well for my role as a mother.

I ultimately decided to return to my former training institution to work off-hours, mainly evenings, so that I could be home during the day with my children while they were young. This has allowed me to be fully present as a mother during most of their waking hours. I have witnessed many milestones achieved and made countless cherished memories I otherwise may have missed had I been working standard business hours.

As my children start preschool and elementary school, I can do most of the school drop-offs and pick-ups that would have conflicted with my prior work schedule. I am familiar with the teachers and staff, and I get to attend various daytime school activities. I am usually home to care for sick children during most of the day and take them to doctor appointments, even at the last minute.

The daytime flexibility is fantastic, but I miss out on family dinnertime and bedtime a few nights a week. Our family capitalizes on the nights I am home, and I have a special time to connect with everyone, even in the evenings I work.

My off-hours schedule is made possible by a supportive spouse. My husband has a job with standard business hours, so he prepares dinners, does bath time, and puts our children to bed in the evenings I work. He is very hands-on with our children and our household tasks. We have made our family life a partnership so that we can maintain fulfilling careers while remaining active and present in our children's lives as they grow. Despite our different schedules, my husband and I try to carve out dedicated time to connect and discuss how our day has gone and what we each missed while away from our children. Having a true partner at home is vital to balancing work and home life.

Having a trusted and reliable caregiver is one of the most critical aspects of balancing a career and family. I am grateful to have family willing and able to provide childcare while my husband and I work. Knowing that our children are safe and loved at work allows me to focus on my radiology work and my patients daily rather than worry about how my children are cared for in my absence. Daycare was fantastic for socialization and novel learning activities in the presence of caring teachers, at the expense of inevitable daycare-associated illnesses. For older children, having afterschool childcare programs and extracurricular activities is very useful, knowing children are safe and having fun with their friends until the workday is done. Many of our friends employ nannies or au pairs for additional help with childcare, transportation, and more.

Though everyone has different career aspirations and trajectories, different family dynamics and needs, and different life circumstances, I offer the following general principles I have learned in my own experience balancing a full-time radiology career and a young family:

Find a job that balances your career goals and your family's needs. These goals and needs will evolve as you and your family grow. Off-hours or night shift positions allow daytime flexibility. Teleradiology is touted as an excellent option for parents of young children, as you can be physically available at home during the workday and save time by not commuting. Part-time work is another means of balancing a career with family life. On-site daycare can be a convenient childcare option, minimizing daily commutes and offering an opportunity to spend time with children during work breaks. Use paid time off to maximize your time with family, whether as extra weeks off during the summer when school is out, time off around special holidays, or even half or full days off at regular intervals.

Regardless of your work schedule, consciously carve out dedicated time for your family. Try to leave work at work during this time, as challenging as it may be. Put away devices and focus on being fully present with your spouse and children. It is not necessarily the quantity of time you have to spend, but how attentive you are to your family when you are with them. If you have the opportunity, consider negotiating more time off rather than monetary benefits since time off is valuable when balancing a career and family.

It truly does take a village, so enlist help however you can. A supportive partner at home can be vital to balancing work and home life. Quality caregivers, whether family, friends, daycare or school staff, nannies, au pairs, or a combination, are also essential. Outsourcing other responsibilities, such as housecleaning, grocery shopping, laundry-related activities, or other house management obligations, can also free up time and energy to devote to family and more enjoyable activities.

Give yourself grace and time to rest. Balancing a career and family is undeniably challenging, especially when each has high demands. Keep sight of your needs, such as sleep, exercise, and hobbies. You need to be at your best to give your best to your family, patients, and colleagues. Remember that this is an evolving process, and we are always a work in progress, but the effort it takes to find a balance between a fulfilling radiology career and a family is well worth it.

Index

J. Shames et al. (eds.), *A Radiologist's Path*,
https://doi.org/10.1007/978-3-031-86882-5